HPNA PALLIATIVE NURSING MANUALS

Pediatric Palliative Care

HPNA PALLIATIVE NURSING MANUALS

Series edited by: Betty R. Ferrell, RN, PhD, MA, FAAN, FPCN, CHPN

Volume 1: Structure and Processes of Care

Volume 2: Physical Aspects of Care: Pain and Gastrointestinal Symptoms

Volume 3: Physical Aspects of Care: Nutritional, Dermatologic, Neurologic, and Other Symptoms

Volume 4: Pediatric Palliative Care

Volume 5: Spiritual, Religious, and Cultural Aspects of Care

Volume 6: Social Aspects of Care

Volume 7: Care of the Patient at the End of Life

Volume 8: Ethical and Legal Aspects of Care

HPNA PALLIATIVE NURSING MANUALS

Pediatric
Palliative Care

Edited by

Betty R. Ferrell, RN, PhD, MA, FAAN, FPCN, CHPN

Professor and Director
Department of Nursing Research and Education
City of Hope Comprehensive Cancer Center
Duarte, California

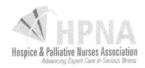

Hospice & Palliative Nurses Association
Advancing Expert Care in Serious Illness

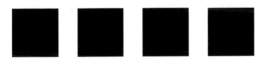

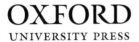

OXFORD
UNIVERSITY PRESS

OXFORD
UNIVERSITY PRESS

Oxford University Press is a department of the University of
Oxford. It furthers the University's objective of excellence in research,
scholarship, and education by publishing worldwide.

Oxford   New York
Auckland   Cape Town   Dar es Salaam   Hong Kong   Karachi
Kuala Lumpur   Madrid   Melbourne   Mexico City   Nairobi
New Delhi   Shanghai   Taipei   Toronto

With offices in
Argentina   Austria   Brazil   Chile   Czech Republic   France   Greece
Guatemala   Hungary   Italy   Japan   Poland   Portugal   Singapore
South Korea   Switzerland   Thailand   Turkey   Ukraine   Vietnam

Oxford is a registered trademark of Oxford University Press
in the UK and certain other countries.

Published in the United States of America by
Oxford University Press
198 Madison Avenue, New York, NY 10016

Library of Congress Cataloging-in-Publication Data
Pediatric palliative care (Ferrell)
Pediatric palliative care/edited by Betty R. Ferrell.
p. ; cm.—(HPNA palliative nursing manuals ; volume 4)
Includes bibliographical references and index.
ISBN 978–0–19–024418–7 (alk. paper)
I. Ferrell, Betty, editor.   II. Hospice and Palliative Nurses Association, issuing body.   III. Title.
IV. Series: HPNA palliative nursing manuals ; v. 4.
[DNLM: 1. Adolescent.   2. Child.   3. Infant.   4. Palliative Care.   5. Hospice and Palliative
Care Nursing-methods.   6. Pediatric Nursing-methods. WS 220]
R726.8
618.92′0029—dc23
2015008132

Contents

Preface   *vii*

Contributors   *ix*

1. Pediatric Hospice and Palliative Care   *1*

    Vanessa Battista and Gwenn LaRagione

2. Symptom Management in Pediatric Palliative Care   25

    Melody Brown Hellsten and Stacey Berg

3. Pediatric Pain: Knowing the Child Before You   47

    Mary Layman Goldstein and Dana Kramer

4. Palliative Care in the Neonatal Intensive Care Unit   69

    Cheryl Thaxton, Brigit Carter, and Chi Dang Hornik

5. Pediatric Care: Transitioning Goals of Care in
    the Emergency Department, Intensive Care Unit,
    and in Between   97

    Barbara Jones, Marcia Levetown, and Melody Brown Hellsten

6. Grief and Bereavement in Pediatric Palliative Care   *121*

    Rana Limbo and Betty Davies

Index   *141*

Preface

This is the fourth volume of a series being published by Oxford University Press in collaboration with the Hospice and Palliative Nurses Association. The intent of this series is to provide palliative care nurses with quick reference guides to each of the key domains of palliative care.

Content for this series was derived primarily from the *Oxford Textbook of Palliative Nursing* (4th edition, 2015) which is also edited by Betty Ferrell, Nessa Coyle, and Judith Paice, the editors of this series. The Contributors identified in each volume are the authors of chapters in the *Oxford Textbook of Palliative Nursing* from which the content was selected for this volume. The *Textbook* contains more extensive content and references, so users of this Palliative Nursing Series are encouraged to use the *Textbook* as an additional resource.

This volume focuses on the area of Pediatric Palliative Care. Chapters address key elements of care for children and families, including pain and symptom management, the provision of hospice and palliative care, and bereavement support for families. This volume also describes settings of pediatric care, including neonatal intensive care, emergency departments, and pediatric intensive care units.

The authors of these chapters are pioneers in the field who have created the models of caring for seriously ill children. There are enormous opportunities to extend palliative care to many other settings of pediatric care, and we hope that this volume can serve as a guide.

Contributors

Vanessa Battista, MS, CPNP, CCRC

Pediatric Nurse Practitioner
The Children's Hospital
    of Philadelphia
Philadelphia, Pennsylvania

Stacey Berg, MD

Professor of Pediatrics
Baylor College of Medicine
    Cancer Center
Texas Children's Cancer Center
Houston, Texas

Brigit Carter, PhD, RN, CCRN

Assistant Professor of Nursing
Duke University Medical Center
Durham, North Carolina

Betty Davies, RN, CT, PhD, FAAN

Adjunct Professor and Senior
    Scholar
School of Nursing
University of Victoria
Victoria, Canada

Mary Layman Goldstein, RN, MS, ANP-BC, ACHPN

Nurse Practitioner
Memorial Sloan-Kettering
    Cancer Center
New York, New York

Melody Brown Hellsten, DNP, RN, PPCNP-BC, CHPPN

Pediatric Nurse Practitioner
Texas Children's Cancer
    Center—PACT
Houston, Texas

Chi Dang Hornik, PharmD, BCPS

Clinical Specialist in Neonatal
    Intensive Care
Department of Pharmacy
Duke University Medical Center
Durham, North Carolina

Barbara Jones, PhD, MSW

Associate Professor of Social Work
Co-Director of The Institute
    for Grief, Loss, and Family
    Survival
The University of Texas at Austin
Austin, Texas

Dana Kramer, RN, MS, FNP-BC

Palliative Medicine NP Fellow
Memorial Sloan-Kettering
    Cancer Center
New York, New York

Gwenn LaRagione, RN, BSN, CCM, CHPPN

Nurse Coordinator
The Children's Hospital
    of Philadelphia
Philadelphia, Pennsylvania

Marcia Levetown, MD, FAAPHM

Principal
HealthCare Communication
    Associates
Houston, Texas

ix

Contributors

Rana Limbo, PhD, RN, PMHCNS-BC, CPLC, FAAN
Associate Director of Resolve Through Sharing
Bereavement and Advance Care Planning Services
Gundersen Health System
La Crosse, Wisconsin

Cheryl Thaxton, RN, MN, CPNP, FNP-BC, CHPPN
Nurse Practitioner—Supportive and Palliative Care Team
Baylor Regional Medical Center at Grapevine
Grapevine, Texas

Chapter 1

Pediatric Hospice and Palliative Care

Vanessa Battista and Gwenn LaRagione

Overview of Pediatric Hospice and Palliative Care

Most societies share a common belief that children symbolize the "future," the dreams and promise of accomplishments yet to be fulfilled. A serious illness or death of an infant, child, or adolescent ("children") generates a threat to such hopes. Bearing witness to these experiences motivates clinicians to do their best to prevent and relieve the suffering of children likely to die, through interventions aimed at cure, and when cure is no longer possible, through interdisciplinary pediatric hospice and palliative care. Pediatric hospice and palliative care nursing requires specialized knowledge, training, and sensitivity to families enduring some of the most arduous moments of their lives. Providing this type of care throughout the illness process, from diagnosis until death, can be simultaneously challenging, physically and emotionally draining, enriching, and meaningful.

Definition of Pediatric Palliative Care

The World Health Organization (WHO) developed one of the earliest and most widely accepted definitions of pediatric palliative care (PPC), describing it as the active total care of the child's body, mind, and spirit, involving an evaluation of a child's psychological, physical, and social distress.[1] That definition has since evolved to include care aimed at improving quality of life of patients facing life-threatening illnesses, and their families, through the prevention and relief of suffering by early identification and treatment of pain and other problems, whether physical, psychological, social, or spiritual.[2] The American Academy of Pediatrics defines PPC as care that should aim to achieve the best quality of life for patients and families, consistent with their values.[3] The Institute of Medicine stated that PPC should consider the needs of patients and families in order to provide timely, accurate, and compassionate information regarding diagnosis, prognosis, and treatment options.[4] PPC can also be defined as both a philosophy of care and an organized, structured system of delivering care to families and children living with life-threatening conditions. The goal of PPC is to prevent and relieve suffering and to maximize quality of life for children of all ages, their family members, and their support systems.

To be practiced effectively, PPC requires an interdisciplinary team (IDT) of professionals from medicine, nursing, psychiatry, psychology, social work, chaplaincy, child life, physical therapy, occupational therapy, speech therapy, art and music therapy, nutrition, pharmacy, and other areas of healthcare (e.g., acupuncturist, massage therapist). PPC offers expert pain and symptom prevention and management and honest discussion about the child's medical condition, which serves as the foundation for collaborative decision-making about goals of care. This patient-focused, family-centered, holistic healthcare should be initiated early in the illness trajectory in support of the child and family to enhance their capacity to cope with a life-threatening condition. PPC aims to preserve the integrity of the family throughout disease progression, addresses anticipatory grief, and provides bereavement support following the death.

Definition and Evolution of Hospice Care

The word *hospice* stems from the Latin *hospes* or *hosptium* meaning "guest house," referring to both guests and hosts, and is thought to have originated in the early 11th century.[4] The National Hospice and Palliative Care Organization (NHPCO) describes hospice as a model of care designed to provide quality compassionate care through a team approach (pain and symptom management and medical, spiritual, and psychosocial care and support) to people with a life-threatening or life-limiting illness. Hospice care focuses on caring for, not curing, the patient while providing support to family, friends, loved ones, and communities.[5]

Comparing Pediatric Palliative and Hospice Care

The terms *palliative care* and *hospice care* are often used interchangeably (as in this chapter) because of their similar core values and philosophical approaches to care. However, it is important to appreciate and understand their main differences. Primarily, palliative care can be provided at any time during the course of the disease (including at the time of diagnosis), whereas hospice care focuses on true end of life care.[6]

Compared with adult care, there are many differences in the provision of pediatric palliative and hospice care. The NHPCO Standards of Practice for Hospice Programs Appendix IV: Pediatric Palliative Care[7] (Table 1.1) provides in-depth insight into these differences. Most notably, children go through developmental stages while having more complex, lifelong chronic conditions, complicating the identification of treatment plans, trajectories, and ethical issues around legal decision-making and all while dealing with larger community involvement, less palliative and hospice care resources, and more complicated grief.[10]

Concurrent Care

When hospice first developed, state and federal regulations and standards governing hospice care and the clinical guidelines for ongoing appropriateness (Medicare and Medicaid) did not address pediatrics. Determining the required 6-months-or-less prognosis was extremely difficult for pediatric physicians because of the wide variability of prognoses in children, often

Table 1.1 Developmental Stages and Perceptions of Death

Age	Basic Conflict	View of Death	Suggestions
Birth to 18 months	Trust vs. mistrust	There is no sense of finality, and death is viewed as continuous with life, reactive to the stress.	Use simple physical communication and provide comforting and nurturing care.
Early childhood to 2 or 3 years	Autonomy vs. shame and doubt	Death is seen as reversible and not final, and the child may feel that death is a punishment. The child may feel responsible for death.	Expect regression, clinging, or aggressive behavior. Encourage expression because the child may be concerned about family function after they die. Use honest and clear language to explain death and dying.
Preschool: 3 to 5 years	Initiative vs. guilt	Death continues to be understood as temporary. The child may have a literal understanding of death and will respond with curiosity and questioning.	Continue to use open communication with clear language. The child should be encouraged to ask questions about death and dying.
School age: 6 to 11 years	Industry vs. inferiority	Death is understood as permanent, and the child understands that the body does not function (no breathing, heart stops beating). The child may also feel responsible and guilty for the illness. The child may have spiritual ideas about afterlife. The child may not want to discuss any feelings.	Reassure the child that death is not his or her fault. Aim to maintain as normal a structure as possible. Include the child in after death plans (funeral planning, last wishes)
Adolescence: 12 to 18 years	Identity vs. role confusion	Adolescents understand the finality of death and may develop a mature understanding of death. They may try to take responsibility for adult concerns within the family (such as finances and caretaking). Feelings of anger may be present.	Allow the time for the child to reflect. Listen to concerns and questions. Support efforts for autonomy and control.

Adapted from Vern-Gross T. Establishing communication within the field of pediatric oncology: A palliative care approach. *Curr Probl Cancer.* 2011;35(6):337-350; and Foster TL, Bell CJ, Gilmer MJ. Symptom management of spiritual suffering in pediatric palliative care. *J Hospice Palliat Nursing.* 2012;14(2):109–115. Table created by Carmen Aguilar Mandac, Columbia University.[8,9]

varying from days to weeks or from months to years. Additionally, referral to hospice care made physicians feel as if they were "giving up" on the children they were treating.

Questions arose as to what—if any—treatments might be acceptable under hospice admission guidelines. Programs varied on whether blood products, antibiotics, infusions, and laboratory tests, for example, were considered "too aggressive" an approach to care, expecting parents to surrender all means of therapies before hospice enrollment. These interventions posed a great financial burden or were unfeasible for many programs, without substantial foundational support. The option of forgoing treatment in order for their child to receive palliative or hospice care was too difficult a decision for parents to make.

Government has since responded by enacting *Concurrent Care for Children* in Section 2302 of the Patient Protection and Affordable Health Care Act (PPACA) on March 23, 2010.[10] This provision allows patients insured by state Medicaid or a Children's Health Insurance Program (CHIP) to receive hospice care while receiving curative treatment. Its ratification demonstrated that healthcare systems and government better understand that the needs of children with life-threatening illnesses or conditions are distinctly different from those of adults.

To better understand and interpret this new act, in 2012, a pediatric-focused Continuum Briefing, *Pediatric Concurrent Care,* was composed at the National Center for Care at the End of Life. This briefing included some barriers to the provision: (1) a physician still needs to certify that the child is expected to die in less than 6 months; (2) every state has different Medicaid-covered services and resources; and (3) the provision itself does not specify what treatments and services are deemed curative.[11] The District of Columbia Pediatric Palliative Care Collaborative and the National Hospice and Palliative Care Organization also recognized these issues and the effort involved for individual states to acclimate and utilize concurrent care. In response, they developed a *Concurrent Care for Children Implementation Toolkit,* designed to guide providers and interested parties in understanding the effect concurrent care would have on their individual state Medicaid programs. It describes how each state has its own amendment and waiver options and encourages learning from other states' experiences to help facilitate a statewide collaborative approach in adapting and implementing effective and efficient concurrent PPC services.[12]

Settings Where Pediatric Palliative Care Occurs

In addition to end of life care, PPC can be implemented in a variety of inpatient and outpatient settings, including acute, chronic, and intensive care units, the emergency department, long-term care facilities, at home, and in schools and communities (Figure 1.1). Because PPC is relatively new, part of the role of the PPC provider is to educate other providers and work to transform the culture in other settings.[13] Many hospitals now have specialized palliative

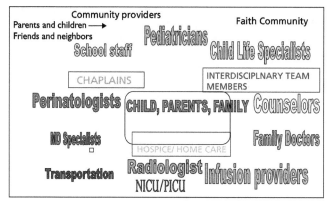

Figure 1.1. Target group for pediatric palliative care.

practices (e.g., the emergency department or the special delivery unit), and some have systems in place in which particular diagnoses generate an automatic referral to the PPC consult service.

Outside the inpatient setting, PPC can take on a variety of different roles. Some hospital-based PPC teams may see patients in the outpatient or clinic setting or may visit with families at home. Also, "if school, service clubs, and faith and various community organizations are a part of the family's social community, and if the family wishes for them to remain an integral part of their life, these organizations should be included as part of the care giving team."[14(p433)] It is essential that PPC teams also liaison with hospice agencies working directly in the home so that families can be better prepared and supported in caring for their children at home, if this is their ultimate goal.

Pediatric Palliative Care and Hospice Service Availability

In evaluating the available outpatient PPC and hospice agencies that care for children, the NHPCO released facts and figures in 2009 (Table 1.2), indicating that of their 4,000 hospice agency members, 10% served pediatric patients through either a dedicated pediatric team or individual staff members trained to care for pediatric patients. Of those 4,000 members, 378 responded to a 2007 survey that provided more in-depth data: 78% reported that they served pediatric patients, with 36% having a pediatric program. For the agencies without a pediatric program, 21.7% had staff members with pediatric experience providing the care or services for children.[13] Additionally, they released data demonstrating the average number of pediatric patients served per year through either PPC or hospice care.

Table 1.2 Outpatient Pediatric Palliative Care and Hospice Agencies Serving Pediatric Patients

Number of Pediatric Patients Served by Agency	Hospice Service	Palliative Care Service
None	14.9%	46.1%
1-10	56.9%	20%
11-20	8%	2.7%
21-50	3.4%	4.1%
51-100	1%	2%
>100	<1%	1.4%
Not reported	12.5%	23.7%

From Friebert S. NHPCO facts and figures: Pediatric palliative and hospice care in America. 2009; http://www.nhpco.org/sites/default/files/public/quality/Pediatric_Facts-Figures.pdf. Accessed April 2, 2015.[15]

Identifying Children Who Could Benefit From Hospice and Palliative Care

The most recent data show that more than 8,600 children need PPC on any given day because of their limited life expectancy and serious healthcare requirements.[15] In the United States, about 50,000 children die annually, but only about 5,000 children receive hospice services each year.[13]

The four generally recognized conditions that lead to death in children are (1) life-threatening conditions for which curative treatment may be feasible but can fail (e.g., cancer, heart disease, trauma or sudden illness, or extreme prematurity); (2) conditions with inevitable premature death, often with long periods of intensive treatment to prolong life and allow participation in normal childhood activities (e.g., cystic fibrosis, human immunodeficiency virus infection, chronic or severe respiratory failure, or muscular dystrophy); (3) progressive conditions without curative treatment options, although children may live several years (e.g., severe metabolic disorders, certain chromosomal disorder, or other rare diseases); and (4) irreversible but nonprogressive conditions with complex healthcare needs leading to complications and likely premature death (e.g., severe cerebral palsy, multiorgan dysfunction, severe pulmonary disability, multiple disabilities following brain or spinal cord infections, or severe brain malformations). A child's illness trajectory can vary greatly depending on age and other factors; overall, the highest rate of death occurs in the first year, with a high proportion occurring in the first month of life.[15]

It is important to recognize that the type and length of a child's illness may affect the timing and ways in which PPC may be implemented (Figure 1.2).[16] They may also affect how family members cope with the child's illness or death and the ways in which they grieve. For example, children in the first group described previously may experience an initial response to treatment, return of disease, and then poor to no response to subsequent treatment. Preoccupation with therapies, laboratory results, or tests may overshadow

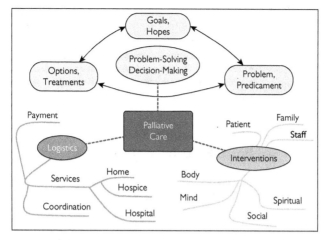

Figure 1.2. Essential elements in pediatric palliative care. (Reprinted with permission from Feudtner C. Collaborative communication in pediatric palliative care: a foundation for problem-solving and decision-making. *Pediatr Clin North Am*. 2007;54[5]:583-607, ix.)

any discussion about the possibility of dying, with the focus instead remaining on managing the disease's medical aspects. Opportunities for comfort may be passed or delayed in the intensive search for cure and life-extending alternatives. PPC may be necessary during periods of prognostic uncertainty, throughout the treatment course, or when treatment fails. In cases of death by trauma or accident, there may be little time to establish relationships, and immediate grief support may be most helpful for the family. Conversely, children with extended and variable pathways through illness, often referred to as *complex chronically ill children*, have multiple peaks and valleys and extensive needs over time. Regardless of the particular condition or disease pathway, accessing PPC can be challenging for all the emotional reasons one might imagine when a child's life is at stake (Figure 1.3).

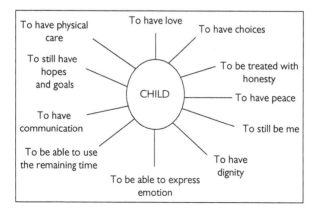

Figure 1.3. Needs of children with life-threatening illness.

The best way to introduce PPC may be to emphasize the philosophy of comprehensive symptom management and simultaneous care for the body, mind, and spirit of both the child and family, while shifting the focus slowly from preserving life to taking measures to relieve suffering and maintain comfort. Nurses are often present for the greatest amount of time and have an extraordinary role in adeptly guiding the family, as well as others members of the IDT, through this emotionally laden course.

Respecting What Parents Want and Need From Healthcare Providers

Nurses can support parents and families in the hospital and at home by identifying their concerns and fears about routine care in the hospital, life outside the security of the hospital, what to expect at home, how to handle emergencies, and when to call for help. Nurses have an important role in creating plans for how they will communicate with the family and in helping families anticipate what may happen in different situations, as well as having appropriate medications, resources, and contacts in place, when needed. In the home setting, parents are the "first responders," and as such, they need adequate access to what is needed to respond best to their child's issues. For example, having an "emergency kit" of a few basic medications in one or two doses for common crisis situations can prevent needless fear and suffering until a home care nurse arrives. Educating parents as thoroughly as possible for transitions in care and settings will reduce anxiety and unnecessary problems at home.

The Interdisciplinary Team

Most PPC teams are composed of physicians, nurse practitioners, nurses, social workers, chaplains, child life specialists, and therapists from different disciplines such as art and music. Some teams may also include nurse coordinators, bereavement coordinators, or psychologists. By definition, "effective palliative care requires a broad multidisciplinary approach that includes the family and makes use of available community resources." PPC IDT members are professionals specially educated and prepared to care for children and families living with life-threatening illness. They can serve as good resources for other allied professionals (e.g., psychiatrists, psychologists, or representatives from other consulting services; primary care providers; physical, occupational, or respiratory therapists; community representatives; teachers, coaches, or religious leaders; and hospice team members), who are also part of a child's care team. Nurses and advanced practice nurses (APNs) may serve as care coordinators as well as liaisons between the child, family, and team (Figure 1.4). Collectively, it is the role of the IDT to accompany the child and family throughout illness, death, and bereavement and to support families in coping with the challenges of living with a life-limiting illness and the suffering that may come along with it.[17]

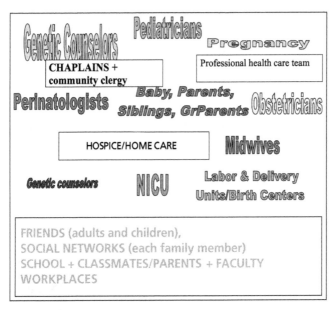

Figure 1.4. Constellation of support and providers. Perinatal palliative care.

Building supportive relationships with families is also a crucial component of effective PPC.[18] Clinicians must be willing to listen and empathize as they build trust with families. Creating an open and nonjudgmental atmosphere and taking a genuine interest in the well-being of a child and family allows for the development of relationships. When IDT members can begin to understand families' beliefs, values, hopes, wishes, expectations, fears, and worries,[19] they can support families in creating goals aligned with what matters most.

Support for Parents and Guardians

Families often describe living with a child with a life-threatening illness as "being on a roller coaster." From the first time a parent senses something is wrong until the time of death, parents are faced with the myriad stressors associated with daily life as well as providing care, making difficult decisions, and often having feelings of guilt or failure.[18] Parents and other family members' needs will range from understanding their child's diagnosis and illness course (informational), to working through feelings of guilt (emotional), to integrating a sense of meaning from the illness experience (meaning-making and spiritual), to support with issues regarding housing, finances, childcare, and work (practical).[18] Parents may feel as if they are losing control over several aspects of their lives, and it is therefore helpful for nurses and other IDT members to find ways to continually allow parents to remain in control, for example, by involving them in planning the child's daily routine, allowing them to participate in care, and asking how they would like things done. The need to feel a sense of control is also relevant to the sick child, who may be fearful from experiencing many physical and emotional changes. Nurses can assist parents with methods to help themselves and their child feel in control of aspects of their experience. Establishing a daily routine, having children participate in conversations about care when appropriate, and knowing what side effects to anticipate from medications, treatments, and therapies foster an environment of mutual trust and respect. Box 1.1 offers some practical advice from a parent's perspective.

Support for Siblings

Caring for the entire family is an essential component of palliative care, and siblings have unique needs. Families will have different opinions regarding sibling involvement, but it is important to consider siblings' psychological, emotional, and social needs and to provide age- and developmentally-appropriate

---

Box 1.1 Family Dynamics: Some Advice From a Parent

Please know that family issues we negotiated as a well family are now under review as a family with a sick child. This is draining and difficult to handle. Therefore, please show patience with us as we struggle to manage an enormous amount of emotional turmoil on many fronts.

Please know that communicating with both parents (if possible) is always far better than each parent separately. Not only does it save you tremendous amounts of time, but even more importantly, it also eliminates the he said/she said issues that can further complicate these emotionally fraught situations.

Please know that we are generally trying our best. Most of us understand the stakes and the issues and are doing our best to deal simultaneously with family issues that have often been problematic for some time.

Please remember that our family communication process may have been ineffective for years and will not improve overnight, even if we recognize that our child needs us now more than ever.

Please know that you are an instrumental part of our family dynamic now and can be of enormous assistance in helping us to heal years of emotional damage due to poor communication.

Please know that we may also be accepting new family members into our lives at this time: stepparents, stepbrothers, and stepsisters, who are also trying to cope with an extraordinarily sensitive situation.

Please know that our difficult family situation may also include issues that do not involve you professionally but that will affect the care of our child, such as divorce, visitation, child support, and custody disputes.

From Levetown M, Meyer EC, Gray D. Communication skills and relational abilities. In: Carter BS, Levetown M, Friebert SE, eds. *Palliative Care for Infants, Children, and Adolescents: A Practical Handbook.* Baltimore: The Johns Hopkins University Press; 2011:169-201. [20]

explanations, as well as opportunities for siblings to be included in aspects of the illness experience.

Strategies for engaging with siblings may be as simple as including siblings during visits (e.g., greeting them by name first when entering a room), asking about their favorite toys or interests, or participating in a small activity together during a home visit. It is important to repeatedly evaluate the well child's level of understanding about the sibling's condition. Family meetings are also a good setting in which to discuss how everyone is doing (including sick and well siblings), how they each perceive the situation, how their needs are or are not being met, and how their fears and concerns can be addressed. The goal for siblings of terminally ill children is to enhance their feelings of involvement from the time of diagnosis to facilitate a healthy adjustment and eventual grieving process.

Interaction With Schools

Children living with complex chronic or life-threatening illnesses may also have an IDT of school caretakers, including teachers, healthcare providers, and therapists (e.g., occupational, speech and language, and physical therapists). Because children spend significant time at school, school personnel are intimately involved in helping meet their various educational, therapeutic, medical, and basic care needs (i.e., feeding, toileting, and hygiene) and play a fundamental role in advocating for them. It is essential to inform school team members of choices families make, especially if those decisions affect the care provided to the child at school. It is also important and helpful to provide education, support, and resources to members of the school team, as well as children's classmates and family members, whenever possible.

Communication

"Let us communicate with each other clearly, compassionately, and collaboratively, as we strive to improve the quality of life for children including, when necessary, that part of life that is dying."[16]

Good communication is the cornerstone of palliative care and serves as the foundation for building and maintaining relationships with families and other team members. Communication serves several purposes, among which are providing and gathering information, expressing sensitivity or empathy, and building partnerships.[20] Having conversations with families about goals of care as early as possible has been shown to reduce suffering.[6] Effective communication allows for an open exchange of information and flow of emotions.[20] It is important to pay attention to subtle verbal and nonverbal cues that may be offered by both children and adult family members. In pediatrics, it is important to ask families whether and how they would like to include their child in discussions, and it is also essential to consider the child's chronologic and developmental age. Effective communication is a skill that must be learned and can be developed over time by all healthcare team members, so that palliative interactions with children, families, and other healthcare team members facilitate "the development of trust, conveyance of compassion, and conduct of ethical decision making." [20(p170)]

Pain and Symptom Management

Pain and symptom management is another essential component of comprehensive and effective PPC because no parent or healthcare provider wishes for children to suffer unnecessarily. Some hospitals have separate pain teams, and many primary teams will manage children's pain and symptoms independently. However, the PPC team may be consulted to recommend a plan, and it is important for nurses to be familiar with general principles of pain and symptom management. Healthcare team members and family members need to be educated about the realities of pain management in children with life-threatening illness and at the end of life.

Nurses who care for children over time will become adept at recognizing when children are in pain or are uncomfortable. In addition, families require practical help, information, explanations, and support. Attention must be paid to the practical issues of preparing for pediatric-appropriate supplies, medications, formulas, feeding tubes, medical equipment, documentation, and teaching tools for parents and children. Ongoing support and education for children and families is an essential part of delivering effective PPC.

Psychological, Emotional, Social, Religious, Spiritual, and Cultural Care

PPC is best delivered by an IDT, including individuals who can provide psychological, social, emotional, and spiritual support, such as psychiatrists, psychologists, social workers, and chaplains. Careful assessment should be conducted regarding the child's and family's developmental level and ability to complete developmental tasks; the experience of emotional symptoms; practical factors, such as financial status, living situation, and social support; and religious, spiritual, or existential background, preferences, beliefs, rituals, and practices.[21] A comprehensive palliative care assessment and plan should include conversations and activities that explore all aspects of children's and families' lives.

Psychological Symptoms and Suffering

It is essential to recognize that the experience of caring for a child with a life-threatening illness may cause family members increased psychological and emotional distress as the illness progresses and the required level of care increases. For example, the extended time required to provide physical care for affected children may result in parents' increased energy expenditures and the feeling that time and energy necessary for other family responsibilities (e.g., other siblings) and activities (e.g., work, community activities) are being depleted. This can also be accompanied by a sense of guilt. The IDT must be alert to the stresses that families endure and routinely talk with them. Although worry and sadness are natural in the context of having or caring for a child with a serious illness, increasing frequency of these symptoms and significant impairment in functioning are signs that the individual or family should be evaluated by a mental health clinician.

It is appropriate for families and children to be offered early psychological and psychiatric consultations to assess the intensity of potential emotional distress because anxiety and depression symptoms are common, treatable, and associated with distress and morbidity, yet are often unrecognized and undertreated in this population of children. Consultations may facilitate open discussions, relationship building, and survival strategies that may help to offset the family's emotional distress.

Anxiety and depression are forms of suffering commonly experienced by children with chronic or life-threatening illnesses and can also encumber the child's primary caregivers, other family members, friends, and siblings. Although there are clear differences in the treatments for anxiety and depression, both disorders are treatable with nonpharmacologic methods. Cognitive-behavioral techniques can be used quite easily by affected children and adults, as well as with medications in conjunction with talk therapy. Examples of nonpharmacologic methods include guided imagery, relaxation and breathing exercises, meditation, reframing automatic negative thoughts, and hypnotherapy (which children can learn to do themselves). Complementary medical therapies, such as physical massage, acupuncture, biofeedback, Reiki, and aromatherapy, can also be extremely helpful in reducing the symptoms of anxiety and depression.

Religious, Spiritual, and Cultural Considerations

Another integral part of providing PPC is an understanding of children's and families' spiritual, religious, and cultural beliefs and how these beliefs influence the decisions they make.[21] The PPC IDT should conduct spiritual assessments with families in a variety of ways because parents of children with serious illness believe that religious or spiritual beliefs are important factors in their coping efforts and decision-making.[21] Chaplains serve to address spiritual suffering, improve family-team communication, and provide rituals that families may request, such as ceremonies or sacraments.[22] Although matters of faith are often discussed with chaplains, any member of the PPC IDT should have some level of comfort in discussing the family's religious and spiritual beliefs, practices, and values. Having these types of discussions may be considered one of the most challenging parts of PPC, but these same discussions may also be some of the most profound, rich, and rewarding.[23] It is therefore important for PPC teams to be open to such discussions and to be aware of and utilize available hospital- and community-based pastoral care services.[21] Table 1.3 provides examples of some open-ended questions to use and

Table 1.3. Examples of Open-Ended Questions to Use and Behaviors to Observe When Assessing Psychosocial Concerns and Strengths in Children and Families

Area Being Assessed	Open-Ended Questions	Patient Behaviors to Observe	Parent Behaviors To Observe
Developmental appropriateness and understanding	• Tell me about what is happening with your treatment. • What questions do you have that you have been too shy or too scared to ask? • Why do you think this is happening to you? (Same questions can be asked of parents.)	• Indications of fearing sleep (will not go to sleep, resists sedative medication) • Indications of fear of separation • Degree to which patient can enjoy some developmentally appropriate activities (artwork, talking to peers, planning fun activities)	• Coddling an older child • Apparent discord between treatment of child and child's developmental level • Ability to let child explore some developmentally appropriate activities • Ability to effectively soothe, nurture, or comfort the child
Beliefs about pain	• What do you think is happening now that is making you hurt? • How worried do you get when you feel pain? What do you worry about? • What do you like (or not like) about using your pain medications? • What concerns do you have about using your patient-controlled analgesia? (Same questions can be asked of parents.)	• Use of a range of physical behaviors to demonstrate different levels of pain • Behavioral manifestations of anxiety with increased pain • Overuse or underuse of pain medications	• Degree of own distress or focus on child's daily pain experience • Ability to comfort and reassure the child • Ability to distract the child from pain and engage in other activities
Emotional issues	• How are you feeling? • What are the things you are sad about? • What are you missing because you are sick? • What are you worried about?	• Sadness, apathy • Lethargy • Unwillingness to engage in activities or conversation (must rule out physical causes for these symptoms)	• Hypervigilance over child's pain, laboratory tests, or physical condition • Signs of anxiety or excess sadness • Avoidance of discussing important issues or of seeing the child or physician • Asking same questions over and over again of the medical team
Communication	• What things would you like to talk or hear about, but haven't been able to find someone to listen or talk to?	• Patient asking questions about death, dying, prognosis, or related issues	• Reluctance to talk to child or to be alone with him or her

	• What opportunities are people offering you to talk, and how does it work if you tell them you don't feel like talking?	• Patient becoming annoyed when people "push" him or her to talk	• Eager insistence that child needs to talk despite child indicating need not to talk • Expressing anger or exaggerated conflicts regarding the medical care
Practical issues	To parents: • How have the extra medical expenses and any lost income you may have experienced affected your family? • How do you get to the hospital for visits? • What meals do you eat when here? • Who is caring for members of the family still at home? • Who lives at home? Who cares for your child when he or she is not in the hospital? • What space is available in your home for hospital equipment? • What would it be like for your family to have home care nursing in the house?	• Missed appointments • Frequently bouncing back to the hospital after discharge • Desire to want to stay in the hospital despite being medically cleared to go home • Strong desire to have no medical intervention (including equipment or home care staff) at home	• Same as child observations
Spiritual needs	• What religious group, if any, do you belong to? • What help would you like in thinking about religious or spiritual issues? • What does your family believe about what happens after death? • What traditions or rituals does your family practice when someone is sick or dying? • What support from the hospital would be most helpful to you?	• Confusion or distress regarding afterlife issues • Worries about what kind of service to have • Unusual behaviors that may be explained or understood as cultural rituals around illness or death	• Same as child observations

Reprinted with permission from McSherry M, Kehoe K, Carroll JM, et al. Psychosocial and spiritual needs of children living with a life-limiting illness. *Pediatr Clin North Am.* 2007;54(5):609–629, ix–x.[21]

behaviors to observe when assessing psychosocial concerns and strengths in children and families and serves as a guideline for having conversations about such topics.

Talking to families about their cultural and ethnic beliefs, customs, and practices is also important and may or may not be tied into their religious or spiritual beliefs. A certified interpreter (i.e., not a family member or other staff member) may be necessary when children and families do not speak English, even if they say they understand what is being said. Various cultures approach children with life-threatening illnesses differently and have beliefs, practices, or rituals surrounding illness and death. It may be unacceptable to speak about illness or death or discuss medical information in front of children. Nurses and other members of the healthcare team should assume a posture of humble curiosity when they do not know the family's culture and customs in depth. Further, it is always important to ask children and families about their personal preferences.

Preserving Hope

A common characteristic of children with life-threatening illness and their families is a prevailing and powerful experience of hope, evidenced in their language and decision-making. It is important to preserve and nurture hope during all stages of the child's illness. No matter how grim the situation, one should always strive to deal with matters in a positive, yet realistic, manner, taking the lead from the child and family. The focus of hope may change over time from hope for cure, to hope for a longer remission than previously, to hope that the child can continue to be cared for at home, to hope that the child will die without pain. Hope may also be centered on a child-specific wish, such as to return to school once more, to celebrate an important birthday, or to celebrate a significant milestone or rite of passage. Other expressions of hope include planning for a visit from grandparents, having friends gathered together, or even gaining the understanding for children, particularly adolescents, that their loved ones will survive and be "okay" after they die. It may become challenging for both families and team members to balance remaining hopeful with realistic expectations. Thus, it is important to openly discuss hopes and fears with children and family members, as well as with other members of the IDT.

Ethical Considerations

A large part of PPC involves helping families with decision-making. Clinical ethical dilemmas are inherent in palliative and end of life care; it will often be the role of the nurse or advanced practice nurse to anticipate, recognize, define, examine, and manage ethically problematic situations[24] that arise in the care of patients and their families. It is important for nurses and IDT team members to be mindful of the potential ethical dilemmas and to be aware of when to consult the hospital's ethics committee for additional support.

Ethical issues that are associated with EOL situations include decision-making under conditions of ambiguity, adequately informing patients and their families about treatment options, balancing quality of life against extending suffering, managing intractable suffering, and futile treatments. Resources are available to help guide the decision-making process and to help children, adolescents, and adults express how they want to be treated throughout their illness and at the time of death from a medical, personal, emotional, and spiritual perspective.[25] Some helpful documents include *My Wishes* (for young children), *Voicing My Choices* (for adolescents), and *Five Wishes* (for adults) published by Aging With Dignity and available at www. agingwithdignity.org.[25]

Care at the Time of Death

Nothing can fully prepare families for the final moments of their loved one's life and the precise time of death, but there is much that can be done to help families anticipate what to expect so as to avoid unnecessary surprises when the time comes. Parents often wonder about these things and may be afraid to ask. Initiating the conversation after a relationship has been established and at a time that feels appropriate is essential. Families should be reminded that PPC clinicians cannot predict exactly when and how death will occur because it can be different for everyone, but parents and family members should be prepared for the possible range of changes that can happen, when they might expect such changes, and what things might look like, feel like, sound like, smell like, and so forth. Consider all the senses for both the adults and any other children who will be present. Parents also may appreciate written hand-outs in language that is not too clinical or frightening so that they may review at a time when they feel ready to do so. Having such knowledge may also prepare parents to talk with each other, other children, and family members.

Children and family members will likely have fears associated with death and the dying process. These may include fears about what dramatic events can unfold, being alone at the time of death, a loved one's missing the death, and being unprepared for an unexpected emergency. Understanding the physical progression of events as death nears and the nearing death awareness that is common among children and adolescents may be reassuring for both members of the team and the family. It is essential to review goals for the time of death well before the time comes so that families feel as in control of the situation as possible. For example, children and families likely will have an idea of where they would like the final hours or days of life to occur, and when possible, nurses and other members of the IDT can try to align the proper resources to allow this to happen. If families desire to remain in the hospital, they should be given a private space or room to be together as a family. Several children's hospitals allocate a specific room or space, often called a "comfort corner," where children may be moved to spend their final hours together with their family. Typically, changing locations close to the end of life is not desired; however, for some families it may be very important to make it home from the hospital or to get to the hospital in the event of an emergency before death. It

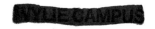

is also crucial to consider whom a family may want present. In most instances, family members will be called to visit as the time of death nears, and the child's bedside, whether in the hospital or at home, can become the gravitational force for loved ones to gather. Families may also have particular wishes about who should be present at the actual moment of death. Sometimes parents want to be alone with their child, with or without other children being present. Other times, families may choose to get in bed with their child. The tenderness and intimacy of these final moments is beyond description, and being present at this time with a family is a very precious privilege for everyone involved in the child's care, especially nurses, who often spend the most time at the bedside and are present during these times.

Creating a Sacred Space

When a child is dying, regardless of age, the very space becomes sacred ground, and it is important to maintain the holiness of that space immediately following the death for even a brief period of time to honor the fact that something very profound has happened (Box 1.2). This allows for a brief pause to honor the nurse's role in maintaining the dignity of a child and his or her family surrounding death before moving on to the next task. Some

Box 1.2 When the Time Comes: How to Help When a Child Dies in the Home—by L.H. Sumner

When the call comes in that a baby or child has died in the home, it may be a challenge and even a bit overwhelming to think of what you will do to be of help and comfort to the grieving family. Below are some guidelines that may help you approach the more prepared and thus more capable of making the process a little less painful for the parents and family.

1. Most parents may not directly ask for a home visit but usually appreciate and often benefit from a visit at the time of the child's death. Just having someone there to help orchestrate the process when they may be feeling overwhelmed and paralyzed by their grief will be helpful. If they refuse, then there are still things to do over the phone that will be helpful for them. It is most likely that they will not need the nurse or other team members to stay for the entire time until the child is taken from the home.

2. Family members should be allowed to have as much time as they need with their baby or child before the mortuary comes to take the child's body. It may seem unusual to you that they would want to keep the body for many hours, but it is a very final step to have their child taken from the home. The mortuary can be notified with the appropriate information required at the time of death but informed that the family will contact them directly when ready.

3. Try to suggest to the parents or caregivers to take some private time alone with the child, without all the family around. This is a very intimate

(continued)

Box 1.2 (Continued)

CHAPTER 1 **Pediatric Hospice and Palliative Care**

19

and personal time for them and may help to facilitate the process of "letting go" and saying goodbye. Others in the family may also wish to have some private time with the child to say a personal goodbye.

4. Encourage the parents and adults present to give any other children in the home or family the *choice* to go in and say goodbye. Children of almost any age are able to decide for themselves if they want to see the child who has died. Just offering children the choice gives them a sense of control during an unfamiliar and unsettling experience. They will remember that someone thought enough of them and their relationship with the person who died to give them the chance to say goodbye. They should be prepared in simple language for what the child will look and feel like. It is a good idea to remove any tubing from infusions, oxygen tubing, catheters, and so forth to normalize the appearance at the bedside as much as possible. Someone the children feels safe with should accompany them. If the family plans on cremation, this may be the last opportunity for them to see their sibling. They may wish to go in for just a "peek," or they may be curious and want to stay around. Whatever length of time they choose to stay is okay and should be up to them.

5. Allow parents to have the time they need to perform any private rituals or activities, which may include bathing the body, redressing the child into something special, rocking the child, or praying at the bedside. They may wish to have their priest, minister, or chaplain come to the home.

6. Suggest to the parents that they may want to save a lock of hair if they have not already done so. They may not feel comfortable doing this themselves and may wish for the staff person to do this. The nape of the neck or the back of the head is the best places to obtain a swatch of hair. It can be tied with a piece of yarn, thread or ribbon. The hair can be placed in an envelope and sealed. Explain that they may not wish to look at it or have it now but that someday they may be glad they had this small remembrance, something tangible that connects them to their loved one, their precious child. A comfortable way to present these suggestions to the family is to say that these are some ideas and suggestions that other parents and families have found to be comforting. They may choose to do all or none of these activities, but the point is to make it meaningful for themselves as a family.

7. There are instances when the family may want to take pictures of the child after death. They may wish to keep them for relatives who live away or for cultural reasons. A family may ask for your assistance to do so, or they may obtain them at the mortuary.

8. If the primary team has not already done so, it may be important to offer the suggestion of taking handprints or footprints of the child. Someone could go out to purchase an ink pad, poster paints, or tempera paints if nothing is available in the home with which to improvise. These supplies are available to the staff in the resource area. Keep a soapy washcloth or alcohol handy to quickly remove the coloring from

(continued)

Box 1.2 (Continued)

the extremity. It is best to try to do the prints as soon as possible before any stiffening of the body sets in. Again, if there are other children in the home, it will be significant to obtain at least one print for the sibling to have for later on. Other family members can add their handprints also, creating a "family portrait" of hands.

9. When contacting the mortuary, emphasize that it was a child who died so that they will be sensitive to the situation they will face. When they arrive at the home, the family may need to say a last goodbye. Rather than have the child taken from the home by the mortuary attendants, we have found that is much less painful if one of the adults or parents carries the child out to the vehicle and surrenders over their child to the arms of the attendants. Parents have told us it felt less traumatic than if they stood back and let the child be *taken* out by "strangers." Occasionally this process becomes an informal processional to accompany the child out of the home for the last time.

10. If at all possible, when the child is ready to be carried out of the home, ask the attendant to keep the child's face and head uncovered and not enclosed completely. The use of the body bag is very distressing and offensive to most parents and family members. Perhaps the child can be wrapped in special blanket or a sheet. Sometimes the driver is willing to take the child partially covered like this until away from the home, and then secure the child's body after leaving the area. Siblings can add a special keepsake to accompany the child's body (e.g., a note, flower, drawing, or stuffed toy).

11. Remind the family of the local bereavement support resources available to them (community or your own organization) and how and when the primary team will be following up. Request that arrangements for a funeral or memorial service be communicated to the child's care team unless it is private, for family only. If visits are made after hours, notify the primary team, including the physicians, of how the family is coping and report on events surrounding the child's death. The primary team can follow up with the child's or sibling's school with permission from the parents.

programs place a special sign on the door, or an image of a dove, butterfly, flower, or leaf, to subtly designate this sacred space and minimize interruptions during this time. Honoring and respecting the space also model to staff that it is not just "business as usual," for a brief time at least. At home, families may choose to have the child remain in his or her bed or keep the space intact for a bit of time before having the body removed. Cultural and religious practices may guide what happens at the time of death and immediately after. Some families may choose to consider organ donation or autopsy, which ideally should be discussed with families before the time of death. If families elect to donate organs or have an autopsy performed, timing will be of the essence, and members of the team and the nurse should be aware of what needs to happen in what timeframe to ensure that a family's wishes are met appropriately.

Self-Care

The team members caring for the child and family will need support before, during, and after the time of death. The nurses present with the family will have other tasks to move on to, but it is very important to have support available to allow for a brief respite, break, or time away from the immediate setting. In some instances, nurses may be given a lighter caseload or, when possible, have time to debrief with another colleague, chaplain, or member of the PPC IDT both immediately and at a later time after the death has occurred. Great wisdom can be shared, burdens lessened, and insights and renewal gained from the time spent debriefing clinically as well as emotionally. It takes a lot of physical, emotional, and psychological energy to care for seriously ill children and members of their family. Preserving the meaning of and sustaining this type of work require self-discipline and intentionality to tend to one's own centering practices and methods of self-care, whether physical, spiritual, or emotional. Self-reflection and self-care, even for a few minutes throughout the day, along with ongoing renewal and reflection outside of work, may be beneficial.

Ongoing professional support from other colleagues is also helpful in sustaining and gaining satisfaction from a career in PPC. Participating in community-based programs, coalitions, professional collaborations, and local and national organizations related to palliative care or pain and symptom management, and teaching or lecturing locally and at professional meetings, are excellent ways to connect with colleagues and develop vital linkages for a thriving PPC program. It is also essential to establish rapport and develop relationships with local colleagues and hospices so that one can comfortably refer families and can work with local community resources to ensure that families get the care they need and deserve.

Anticipatory Grief and Bereavement

Children and families often begin the process of anticipatory grief at the time of diagnosis, and it is helpful for PPC team members to talk with children and families continually about the ongoing losses that they are experiencing. Grief continues through and beyond the time of death, and families, community members, and team members who cared for the child and family will need ongoing bereavement support. Many hospitals have at least annual ceremonial remembrance services that families and team members find helpful for honoring and remembering the children who have died.

Overview of Nursing Care Issues for Pediatric Palliative Care

The responsibilities of caring for children living with life-threatening illnesses and their families are extensive and require an understanding of the interconnectedness of the myriad aspects of illness and suffering: physical, emotional, psychological, spiritual, and social. Illness unravels the pattern that belongs uniquely to each child, interrupting the ongoing stories of children's lives. Nurses and members of the PPC IDT must assess for imbalances and indications of suffering in each of these areas to appropriately intervene and provide comprehensive and effective PPC.

Education and Training

In recognizing that hospice and palliative nursing care has become a specialized area of nursing, the Hospice and Palliative Nurses Association (HPNA) was established in 1986. This membership organization relies on evidence-based research and data to assist members in delivering quality nursing care, symptom management, grief and bereavement support, guidance with difficult conversations, education, and encouragement in leadership and mentoring efforts. The HPNA supports credentialing for advanced practice registered nurses, adult and pediatric registered nurses, licensed practical nurses, licensed vocational nurses, nursing assistants, and administrators through the National Board for Certification of Hospice and Palliative Nurses (NBCHPN).[26]

Additionally, recognizing that nurses need specialized training in hospice and PPC, many professional associations are supporting localized efforts by cosponsoring educational efforts with other entities such as the well-established and respected End-of-Life Nursing Education Consortium (ELNEC). ELNEC is a national education initiative to improve palliative care by teaching nurses at all levels about PPC, so that they can teach this essential information to nursing students and other practicing nurses.[27] Updated annually, the pediatric curriculum includes 10 learning modules that highlight current practices and include cases, key references, supplemental teaching tools, and resources. A new curriculum for advanced practice nurses, launched by ELNEC in 2012, also includes pediatric-specific training modules. Although too numerous to list completely, several national professional organizations offer specific training in both adult and pediatric palliative care for healthcare providers in all disciplines. The Center to Advance Palliative Care (CAPC) provides healthcare professionals with the tools, training, and technical assistance necessary to start and sustain palliative care programs in hospitals and other settings and includes an extensive listing of other trainings that are available on their website (http://www.capc.org). The Initiative for Pediatric Palliative Care (IPPC), sponsored by the Educational Development Center (EDC), is an interdisciplinary model of case-based experiential training that offers PPC-specific training events. More information and additional training materials can be found at the IPPC website (www/ippcweb.org). The National Hospice and Palliative Care Organization (NHPCO)[10] also has developed a pediatric curriculum to address the ongoing demand for training of adult hospice programs to be prepared to care for children (http://www.nhpco.org). In short, there are an increasing number of educational offerings and opportunities for nurses and other healthcare professionals to expand their burgeoning knowledge of PPC.

Acknowledgment

The authors gratefully acknowledge Lizabeth H. Sumner for her original work and ongoing contributions.

References

1. World Health Organization. WHO definition of pediatric palliative care. 1998; http://www.who.int/cancer/palliative/definition/en/. Accessed April 2, 2015.

2. American Academy of Pediatrics Committee on Bioethics and Committee on Hospital Care. Palliative care for children. 2000; http://pediatrics.aappublications.org/content/106/2/351.full. Accessed April 25, 2015.

3. American Academy of Pediatrics Committee on Bioethics and Committee on Hospital Care. Palliative care for children. *Pediatrics.* 2000;106(2):351-57.

4. Wikipedia, the Free Encyclopedia. Hospice. Linguistically, the word "hospice" derives from the Latin hospes, a word which ... Historians believe the first hospices originated in the 11th century, around 1065. http://en.wikipedia.org/wiki/Hospice. Accessed April 24, 2015.

5. National Hospice and Palliative Care Organization. Hospice Care. 2013; http://www.nhpco.org/about/hospice-and-palliative-care. Accessed April 2, 2015.

6. Crozier F, Hancock LE. Pediatric palliative care: beyond the end of life. *Pediatr Nurs.* 2012;38(4):198–203, 227; quiz 204.

7. National Hospice and Palliative Care Organization. Standards of Practice for Hospice Programs. Appendix VI PPC PFC 1: Pediatric Palliative Care (PPC PFC). 2012; http://www.nhpco.org/sites/default/files/public/quality/Standards/APXIV.pdf. Accessed April 2, 2015.

8. Vern-Gross T. Establishing communication within the field of pediatric oncology: a palliative care approach. *Curr Probl Cancer.* 2011;35(6):337-350.

9. Foster TL, Bell CJ, Gilmer MJ. Symptom management of spiritual suffering in pediatric palliative care. *J Hospice Palliat Nurs.* 2012;14(2):109-115.

10. Office of the Legislative Counsel. Compilation of Patient Protection and Affordable Care Act, As Amended Through May 1, 2010 Including Patient Protection and Affordable Care Act Health-Related Portions of the Health Care and Education Reconciliation Act of 2010. Vol. 1112012:202-203.

11. National Hospice and Palliative Care Organization. Pediatric palliative care. 2012; http://www.nhpco.org/resources/pediatric-hospice-and-palliative-care. Accessed April 2, 2015.

12. District of Columbia Pediatric Palliative Care Collaboration & National Hospice and Palliative Care Organization. Concurrent Care for Children Implementation Toolkit, Section 2302 of the Patient Protection and Affordable Care Act. 2013; http://www.nhpco.org/sites/default/files/public/ChiPPS/CCCR_Toolkit.pdf. Accessed April 2, 2015.

13. Weise K, Levetown M, Tuttle C, Liben S. Palliative care in the pediatric intensive care setting. In: Carter BS, Levetown M, Friebert SE, eds. *Palliative Care for Infants, Children, and Adolescents: A Practical Handbook.* Baltimore: The Johns Hopkins University Press; 2011:387-413.

14. Huff SM, Orloff SF, Wheeler J, Grimes L. Palliative care in the home, school, and community. In: Carter BS, Levetown M, Friebert SE, eds. *Palliative Care for*

Infants, Children, and Adolescents: A Practical Handbook. Baltimore: The Johns Hopkins University Press; 2011:414-440.

15. Friebert S. NHPCO facts and figures: pediatric palliative and hospice care in America. 2009; http://www.nhpco.org/sites/default/files/public/quality/Pediatric_Facts-Figures.pdf. Accessed April 2, 2015.

16. Feudtner C. Collaborative communication in pediatric palliative care: a foundation for problem-solving and decision-making. *Pediatr Clin North Am.* 2007;54(5):583-607, ix.

17. Papadatou D, Bluebond-Langner M, Goldman A. The team. In: Wolfe J, Hinds PS, Sourkes BM, eds. *Textbook of Interdisciplinary Pediatric Palliative Care.* Philadelphia: Elsevier Saunders; 2011:55-63.

18. Jones BL, Gilmer M, Parker-Raley J, et al. Parent and sibling relationships and the family experience. In: Wolfe J, Hinds PS, Sourkes BM, eds. *Textbook of Interdisciplinary Pediatric Palliative Care.* Philadelphia: Elsevier Saunders; 2011:135-147.

19. Kane JR, Joselow M, Duncan J. Understanding the illness experience and providing anticipatory guidance. In: Wolfe J, Hinds PS, Sourkes BM, eds. *Textbook of Interdisciplinary Pediatric Palliative Care* Philadelphia: Elsevier Saunders; 2011:30-40.

20. Levetown M, Meyer EC, Gray D. Communication skills and relational abilities. In: Carter BS, Levetown M, Friebert SE, eds. *Palliative Care for Infants, Children, and Adolescents: A Practical Handbook.* Baltimore: The Johns Hopkins University Press; 2011:169-201.

21. McSherry M, Kehoe K, Carroll JM, et al. Psychosocial and spiritual needs of children living with a life-limiting illness. *Pediatr Clin North Am.* 2007;54(5):609-629, ix-x.

22. Fitchett G, Lyndes KA, Cadge W, et al. The role of professional chaplains on pediatric palliative care teams: perspectives from physicians and chaplains. *J Palliat Med.* 2011;14(6):704-707.

23. Lanctot D, Morrison W, Kock KD, Feudtner C. Spiritual dimensions. In: Carter BS, Levetown M, Friebert SE, eds. *Palliative Care for Infants, Children, and Adolescents: A Practical Handbook.* Baltimore: The Johns Hopkins University Press; 2011:227-243.

24. Kirschen MP, Feudtner C. Ethical issues. In: N. S. Abend & M. A. Helfaer, eds. *Pediatric Neurocritical Care.* New York: DemosMedical; 2013:485-493.

25. Aging with dignity: my wishes, voicing my choices, and five wishes. 2012; http://www.agingwithdignity.org/index.php. Accessed April 2, 2015.

26. Hospice and Palliative Nursing Association. About us and certification info. 2013; http://www.hpna.org/Default2.aspx. Accessed April 2, 2015.

27. End-of-Life Nursing Education Consortium (ELNEC). 2013; http://www.aacn.nche.edu/elnec. Accessed April 2, 2015.

Chapter 2

Symptom Management in Pediatric Palliative Care

Melody Brown Hellsten and Stacey Berg

Complex chronic conditions of childhood (Box 2.1) are medically defined as "any medical condition that can be reasonably expected to last at least 12 months, involves either multiple organs or one organ system severely enough to require specialty pediatric care, and some probability of hospitalization at a tertiary care center."[1] A needs-based definition of children with complex chronic conditions includes "children who require ongoing skilled monitoring and care from family or professional caregivers and use supportive therapies and technology to enhance health and well-being to avert death or further disability."[2]

Ongoing advances in medical science are contributing to life-prolonging management of children with complex chronic conditions. However, this life prolongation often comes at the cost of multiple acute and chronic health crises and hospitalizations.[3] Worsening debilitation, as the child's condition progresses, increases the likelihood of suffering for the child and family.[3,4] It is, therefore, imperative that care providers face the challenge of recognizing and attending to suffering as a concurrent focus of care, while providing curative and life-prolonging treatment.

Assessing Sources of Suffering in Advanced Childhood Illness

Illness Experience and Sources of Suffering

Research exploring the experiences of families of children with complex chronic conditions provides a glimpse into their world. Uncertainty prevails as the parents move from the initial suspicion that something is wrong with their child to the confirmation that this is indeed the case.[5-8] Parents struggle to cope with the diagnosis and learn skills necessary to provide technical care and negotiate the care system for needed services and information. Over time, parents must live with ongoing uncertainty regarding the unpredictability of the illness, the ultimate outcome of their child's treatment, the challenges of parenting a seriously ill child, and the possibility of death.[9-12] The child may experience disability, physical pain, and other distressing symptoms as a result of the disease and treatments, severe alterations in their social world, and

Box 2.1 Categories of Complex Chronic Conditions of Childhood

Neurologic Conditions

Congenital malformations of the brain
Anencephaly
Lissencephaly
Holoprosencephaly
Cerebral palsy and mental retardation

Neurodegenerative Disorders

Muscular dystrophies
Spinal muscular atrophy
Adrenoleukodystrophy
Epilepsy

Cardiovascular Conditions

Malformations of the heart and great vessels
Cardiomyopathies
Conduction disorders and dysrhythmias

Respiratory Conditions

Cystic fibrosis
Chronic respiratory disease
Respiratory malformations

Renal Conditions

Chronic renal failure

Gastrointestinal Conditions

Congenital anomalies
Chronic liver disease and cirrhosis
Inflammatory bowel disease

Hematologic and Immunodeficiency Conditions

Sickle cell disease
Hereditary anemias
Hereditary immunodeficiency
HIV/AIDS

Metabolic Conditions

Amino acid metabolism
Carbohydrate metabolism
Mucopolysaccharidosis
Storage disorders

Genetic Conditions

Trisomy 18
Chromosome 22 deletions
Other congenital disorders

Malignancy

Leukemias and lymphomas
Brain tumors
Sarcomas
Neuroblastoma

disruption of their developmental process.[4] Siblings may experience feelings of anger, guilt, anxiety, depression, and social isolation.[13]

Assessing and understanding the child and family's unique experiences during the illness trajectory provides the care team with insight into what symptoms may contribute to the family's suffering. This assessment involves hearing the child's and family members' "story" as they have lived it, during the course of the disease. It is important to elicit care that was helpful in past experiences as well as care that was not helpful. Insights into what the family values regarding the role of spirituality or faith, the meaning they give to their illness experience, and what activities or interactions the child and family identify as contributing to quality of life provide a context for identifying and managing symptoms that contribute to the child's and family's suffering.

Expectations and Goals of Care

Goals of care for children with serious, life-threatening, or limiting illness include interventions aimed at cure; life prolongation, with or without aggressive life-sustaining therapies; and care focused solely on treating discomfort from symptoms as the disease moves into its terminal phase. Ideally, these goals will shift as the child, family, and primary healthcare team discuss changes in quality of life, symptoms, and prognosis over the disease trajectory. It is very important that interventions aimed at maintaining maximal comfort and quality of life occur throughout the disease trajectory, as well as through the terminal stages. Conversely, the presence of a do-not-resuscitate (DNR) order should not lead to healthcare professionals' dismissing treatable illnesses or symptoms as "part of the dying process," contributing to child and family suffering.

The parents' most difficult decision is to change the focus of care from cure or aggressive life prolongation to comfort and terminal care. In 2000, Wolfe and colleague[14] drew attention to symptoms and suffering experienced by children with cancer, as well as to the disparity between parents and care providers regarding the realization that a child with progressive cancer had no realistic chance for cure. Parents who came to that realization earlier were more likely to discuss hospice care, establish a DNR order, and change the focus of care from cancer-directed therapies to treatments controlling discomfort and an increased perception of quality care at home. Parents have reported that decisions to forgo further aggressive medical treatments and, instead, to pursue care focused on comfort and quality of life occurred only after realizing that ongoing aggressive treatment would not bring about cure or further life prolongation and recognizing the physical deterioration and suffering of their child. After this realization is reached, parents report that the child's wishes and quality of life are major determinants of treatment decision-making.[11]

The first step to managing symptoms of children with advanced and terminal illness is a thorough assessment of the child's and family's expectations and goals of care. Interventions aimed at controlling symptoms must be compatible with the family's understanding of where their child is in the disease trajectory and their expectations of care, as well as the child's overall functional status and quality of life. In determining the expectations and goals of care with the child and family, it is important to discuss the balance between relieving and contributing to the child's suffering. The prevailing decision-making framework should be based not on whether an intervention is consistent with a palliative care focus but, rather, on whether the intervention would provide relief from or contribute to the child's and family's suffering.

Physical Symptoms and Suffering

Children dying as the result of complex chronic conditions experience numerous symptoms throughout their illness trajectory that can contribute to suffering and decreased quality of life. (Box 2.2). Assessment should include the child's report of symptoms and how distressing he or she finds them, information based on parent observation of their child's condition, and the healthcare provider's knowledge of the pathophysiology of the underlying disease. Diagnostic tests should be considered carefully for the potential discomfort they may cause. Tests should be ordered only if they will help determine an intervention. A test's appropriateness should be questioned if its results will not change management (e.g., magnetic resonance imaging to document growth of known terminal tumor).

Control of present symptoms and anticipation of distressing symptoms, as disease progresses, are imperative in attending to the suffering of children with advanced disease. Following is a discussion of the most common symptoms associated with distress and suffering, experienced by children with advanced illness. Starting dosages of medications will vary depending on the

---

Box 2.2 Symptoms Contributing to Suffering in Advanced and Terminal Disease

General Symptoms

Fatigue

Anorexia

Psychological and Emotional Symptoms

Anxiety and depression

Neurologic Symptoms

Seizures

Somnolence

Respiratory Symptoms

Dyspnea

Gastrointestinal Symptoms

Nausea and vomiting

Constipation

Diarrhea

age, weight, and clinical circumstances of the child. It is incumbent on physicians and nurses to consult with experienced pediatricians and pediatric hospice and palliative care providers for medication choices, appropriate doses, and titration for difficult cases of symptom management.

Fatigue

The most comprehensive research in fatigue experienced by children with complex chronic illnesses has been in the area of childhood cancer. Fatigue has been described as a "profound sense of being physically tired, or having difficulty with body movements such as moving legs or opening their eyes" in young children with cancer and as a "changing state of exhaustion that includes physical, mental, and emotional tiredness" in adolescents with cancer.[14] Fatigue, lethargy, lack of energy, and drowsiness have been reported in more than 50% of children with cancer and have been described as moderately to severely distressing.[15]

Fatigue is a multidimensional symptom that can be related to disease, treatment, or emotional factors (Box 2.3). Assessment requires a multidimensional approach, which includes subjective and objective data to determine the degree of distress and potential causes of the child's fatigue. Subjective assessment involves asking children about their feelings of tiredness or lack of energy, how long they feel tired, when they feel most tired, and how it affects their ability to play or go to school. Objective assessment should include vital signs, presence of other symptoms such as dyspnea or vomiting, evaluation of hydration status, and muscle strength. Laboratory data may include parameters such as oxygen saturation, complete blood count and differential, and thyroid studies. Management of fatigue will vary depending on the underlying cause and may include both pharmacologic and nonpharmacologic interventions (Table 2.1).

Box 2.3 Factors Contributing to Fatigue in Children With Advanced Disease

Disease and treatment
Pain
Unresolved symptoms
Anemia
Malnutrition
Infection
Fever
Sleep disturbance
Debilitation
Psychological factors
Depression
Anxiety
Spiritual distress
Management of symptoms during disease progression and end of life
General systemic symptoms

Table 2.1 Management of Fatigue in Children With Advanced Disease

Cause	Intervention	Dose	Comments
Pharmacologic Management			
Anemia	Blood transfusion	10–15 mL/kg IV over 4 h	Premedicate with diphenhydramine (1 mg/kg/ IV/PO, max dose 50 mg), acetaminophen (10–15 mg/ kg PO) and hydrocortisone (2 mg/kg IV, max dose 100 mg) before transfusion if history of reaction.
Psychostimulants			
Disease progression	• Methyl- phenidate	0.3 mg/kg/ dose PO bid	Dosage information for ≥6 y. Give doses in a.m. and early afternoon. May titrate by 0.1 mg/kg/dose to max of 2 mg/kg/day, gauge by child's desired activity level. May decrease appetite
	• Dextroam- phetamine	6–12 y: 5 mg/day May titrate in 5-mg increments weekly 12 y: 10 mg/day	Titrate according to child's desired level of activity. Will suppress appetite
Sleep Agents			
Insomnia, anxiety			
	• Diphen- hydramine	1 mg/kg IV/PO Max dose 50 mg/dose	May cause paradoxical excitement, euphoria, or confusion
			May use in children as young as 2 y
	• Lorazepam	0.03–0.1 mg IV/PO. Max 2 mg/dose	Can cause retrograde amnesia. Taper dose with prolonged use.
			May use in infants and young children
	• Zolpidem	10 mg PO qh	Use for adolescents, young adults. No dosing information in young children.
Nonpharmacologic Management			
Anorexia	Nutritional supplementation (e.g., Boost, Pediasure)		

(continued)

Table 2.1 (Continued)	
Generalized fatigue all causes	Frequent rest, energy conservation
Deconditioning, weakness	Physical/ occupational therapies
All causes	Play therapy
All causes	Exploring fears and anxiety that may interfere with sleep

From Ullrich CK, Mayer OH. Assessment and management of fatigue and dyspnea in pediatric palliative care. *Pediatr Clin North Am*. 2007;54(5):735–756.[16]

Nausea and Vomiting

The pathophysiology of nausea and vomiting can be acute, anticipatory, or delayed; requires careful assessment to determine underlying causes; and can cause extreme exhaustion and dehydration, if not well controlled. Underlying causes may include decreased gastric motility, constipation, obstruction, metabolic disturbances, medication side effects or toxicity, and increased intracranial pressure.

A detailed assessment of the onset, duration, and concomitant symptoms (e.g., headache, visual disturbances) must be obtained. Medical management of nausea and vomiting is based on the suspected underlying cause (Table 2.2).

Corticosteroids may be helpful in reducing an intestinal obstruction. Antiemetic medications, combined with medications to reduce secretions (e.g., glycopyrrolate), can be helpful in relieving nausea and vomiting related to intestinal obstruction. In cases of severe nausea and vomiting related to obstruction, placement of a nasogastric tube can decompress the stomach and provide comfort. Medications that promote gastric emptying (e.g., metoclopramide) or motility should not be used, if obstruction is suspected. Steroids can provide relief from vomiting caused by increased intracranial pressure. Nausea and vomiting related to medications or anorexia may be managed by a number of antiemetic medications.[18,19] Relaxation techniques, deep breathing, distraction, and art therapies may assist in reducing anticipatory nausea.

Constipation

Constipation is a frequent symptom experienced by children with advanced and terminal illness and can occur even in children with limited oral intake. Children and adolescents, in particular, become embarrassed if asked about bowel habits and will deny problems, leading to a severe problem. It is important to educate the child and family about the potential distress constipation can cause and determine how to discuss this issue. Constipation occurs as a result of inactivity, dehydration, electrolyte imbalance, bowel compression

Table 2.2 Management of Nausea and Vomiting

Agent	Dose	Comments
Ondansetron	0.15 mg/kg/dose IV or 0.2 mg/kg dose PO q4h; max: 8 mg/dose	Indicated for opioid-induced nausea/vomiting
Metoclopramide	1–2 mg/kg/dose IV q2–4h; max: 50 mg/dose	Indicated for nausea/vomiting related to anorexia, gastroesophageal reflux
		Can cause dystonia
Promethazine	0.5 mg/kg IV/PO q4–6h; max: 25 mg/dose	Indicated for nausea/vomiting related to obstruction, opioids. May increase sedation
Dexamethasone	1–2 mg/kg IV/PO initially, then 1–1.5 mg/kg/day divided q6h; max: 16 mg/day	Indicated for nausea/vomiting related to bowel obstruction, intracranial pressure, medications
		Side effects include weight gain, edema, and gastrointestinal irritation

Adapted from Karwacki MW. Gastrointestinal symptoms. In: Goldman A, Hain R, Liben S, eds. *Oxford Textbook of Palliative Care for Children.* London and New York: Oxford University Press; 2006:342–372.[17]

or invasion by tumor, nerve involvement, or medications. Symptoms include anorexia, nausea, vomiting, colicky abdominal pain, bloating, and fecal impaction. Physical examination may reveal abdominal distention, right lower-quadrant tenderness, and fecal masses. A rectal examination should be done; however, it is important to gain the child's or adolescent's trust before such an invasive assessment. Ask the child which parent he or she would prefer to be present and have that parent sit near the child and provide reassurance and comfort. Assess the rectum for presence of hard impacted feces, an empty dilated rectum, or extrinsic compression of the rectum by a tumor, hemorrhoids, fissures, tears, or fistulas. Caution should be used in children with cancer who are neutropenic, and a digital examination should not be done unless absolutely necessary.

Management is aimed at preventing constipation from occurring, but if constipation has occurred, it should be treated immediately to avoid debilitating effects (Box 2.4). Stool softeners should be given for any child at risk for constipation caused by opioid pain management or decreased activity. Softeners are most effective when children are well hydrated, so the healthcare provider should encourage the child to drink water, as tolerated. Stimulant laxatives should be used if a child has not had a bowel movement for more than 3 days past that child's usual pattern. If these measures are not successful, stronger cathartic laxatives (e.g., magnesium citrate) or an enema may be used. If there is stool in the rectum and the child is unable to pass it, digital disimpaction may be necessary. The child should be prepared for the procedure and premedicated with pain and antianxiety medications.

Box 2.4 Management of Constipation

Senna

Infants and children <12 y

Syrup:

1 mo to <2 y: 1.25–2.5 mL (2.2–4.4 mg sennosides) at bedtime [max: 2.5 mL (4.4 mg sennosides) twice daily]

2 to <6 y: 2.5–3.75 mL (4.4–6.6 mg sennosides) at bedtime [max: 3.75 mL (6.6 mg sennosides) twice daily]

6 to <12 y: 5–7.5 mL (8.8–13.2 mg sennosides) at bedtime [max: 7.5 mL (13.2 mg sennosides) twice daily]

Tablet:

2 to <6 y: 1/2 tablet (4.3 mg sennosides) at bedtime [max: 1 tablet (8.6 mg sennosides) twice daily]

6 to <12 y: 1 tablet (8.6 mg sennosides) at bedtime [max: 2 tablets (17.2 mg sennosides) twice daily]

Children ≥12 y and Adults

Syrup: 10–15 mL (17.6–26.4 mg sennosides) at bedtime [max: 15 mL (26.4 mg sennosides) twice daily]

Tablet: 2 tablets (17.2 mg sennosides) at bedtime [max: 4 tablets (34.4 mg sennosides) twice daily]

Ducosate Sodium

Children < 3 y: 10–40 mg/day PO in 1–4 divided doses

3–6 y: 20–60 mg/day PO in 1–4 divided doses

6–12 y: 50–150 mg/day PO in 1–4 divided doses

>12 y: 50–100 mg/day PO in 1–4 divided doses

Diarrhea

Although diarrhea is far less common in children with terminal illnesses, it still may occur and contribute to a diminished quality of life. Diarrhea may be caused by intermittent bowel obstruction, fecal impaction, medications, malabsorption, infections, history of abdominal or pelvic radiation, chemotherapy, inflammatory bowel disease, and foods with sorbitol and fructose (found frequently in juices, gum, and candy). Diseases related to increased risk for diarrhea include HIV/AIDS resulting from infections, cystic fibrosis related to malabsorption, and malignancies related to disease progression and treatment history.

Assessment should include onset, suddenness, duration, and frequency of loose stools; incontinence; character of the stools (color, odor, consistency, presence of mucus or blood), bowel sounds, presence of palpable masses or feces, abdominal tenderness, and examination of the rectal area. Assessment of dehydration includes observation of mucous membranes for dryness, cracking, poor skin turgor, and generalized fatigue.

Diet and medication history should be reviewed for potential causes of diarrhea.

Treatment is aimed at managing the underlying causes and the results of persistent diarrhea (Box 2.5). Dietary intervention should involve continued feeding of the child's regular diet as tolerated, as well as oral rehydration with electrolyte solutions as tolerated. For debilitated children using incontinence garments, attention to skin condition and prevention of breakdown is imperative.

Feeding Problems and Intolerance

Gastrointestinal symptoms and related feeding problems are common in children with neurologic impairments. Oropharyngeal dysphagia, gastroesophageal reflux, dysmotility, retching or vomiting, aspiration, and constipation represent a common cluster of symptoms of children with both static and progressive neurologic impairment.[20,21] Symptom management is focused on balancing treatment of the underlying complications as well as the child's nutritional needs.[22,23] For children with mild forms of neurologic impairment, oromotor stimulation and feeding therapy can be helpful in maintaining nutrition.[24] For children with severe or progressive neurologic conditions, malnutrition and aspiration risk complicate oral feeding. Gastrostomy tubes can improve nutrition, medication delivery, and caregiver stress around feeding, but do not necessarily improve the patient's overall quality of life.[21,25] A retrospective review of fundoplication and gastrojejunal feeding tubes for prevention of aspiration pneumonia found neither option superior for preventing aspiration pneumonia or improving overall survival.[26]

Anorexia and Cachexia

Loss of appetite occurs in nearly all children with terminal illness. Anorexia involves the loss of desire to eat or a loss of appetite, with associated decrease in food intake. Cachexia is a general lack of nutrition and wasting

---

Box 2.5 Management of Diarrhea

Loperamide

Initial doses: 2–5 y: 1 mg PO tid;

6–8 y: 2 mg PO bid;

8–12 y: 2 mg PO tid; after initial dose, 0.1-mg/kg doses after each loose stool (not to exceed the initial dose);

>12 y: 4 mg PO × 1 dose; then 2 mg PO after each loose stool (max: 16 mg/day)

Diphenoxylate and Atropine

2–5 y: 2 mg PO tid (not to exceed 6 mg/day)

5–8 y: 2 mg PO qid (not to exceed 8 mg/day)

8–12 y: 2 mg PO 5 times/day (not to exceed 10 mg/day)

>12 y: 2.5–5 mg PO 2–4 times/day (not to exceed 20 mg/day)

of lean muscle mass that occurs over the course of a chronic progressive disease. Anorexia and cachexia are multidimensional in nature, influenced by disease, treatment, and emotional factors.[27,28] (Box 2.6). These symptoms are particularly distressing to parents of children with illness because they fear the child is "starving to death." Food and meals have a social association with "caring" and are significant in family culture, activities, and ritual. In most instances, children will request favorite foods, as a means of comfort and familiarity. It is important to assist parents in understanding their child's changing eating habits and nutritional needs, and how to redirect energies toward other caregiving activities. Table 2.3 provides additional suggestions for management of anorexia and cachexia.

Aggressive nutritional support does not usually improve the condition and may add additional symptom burden for the child. When the family chooses medically provided nutritional interventions, the challenge is balancing fluid and nutritional supplementation because appetite and metabolic needs decrease with advancing disease. Complication rates for enteral feeds are upward of 76% and include fluid overload, electrolyte imbalance, pain, nausea, and vomiting.[30]

Ideally, as the child's condition progresses, parenteral or enteral supplements can be slowly weaned to promote comfort and decrease symptoms of increased congestion or secretions.

Anxiety

Children with chronic illness may experience numerous anxiety-provoking events. Serious illness, hospitalizations, painful procedures, changes in independence and physical abilities, uncontrolled pain and other symptoms, and an uncertain future all can contribute to fear and anxiety. The distinction between childhood fears and anxiety is crucial—childhood fears

---

Box 2.6 Factors Contributing to Anorexia and Cachexia in Advanced Disease

Physiologic Factors

Uncontrolled pain or other symptoms
Feeding and swallowing problems
Poor oral hygiene and infections
Mouth sores
Nausea and vomiting
Constipation
Delayed gastric emptying
Changes in taste

Psychological Factors

Depression
Anger
Stress
Psychological and emotional symptoms

Table 2.3 Management of Anorexia and Cachexia

Intervention	Dose	Comments
Pharmacologic Management		
Megestrol	10 mg/kg/ dose PO bid	May cause headache, rash, hypertension
Dronabinol	2.5 mg/kg/ dose 3–4 times/day	Provides triple effect of antiemetic, appetite stimulant, mood elevation. May be used in young children
Nonpharmacologic Management		
Prepare small portions of favorite foods.		
Allow child to eat "comfort" foods, don't stress "balanced diet."		
Use thickened liquids or soft foods.		
Offer shakes, smoothies, and other high-calorie foods.		
Provide nutritional drinks as tolerated.		
Assist family in limiting stress over child's eating.		

From Santucci G, Mack JW. Common gastrointestinal symptoms in pediatric care: nausea, vomiting, constipation, anorexia, cachexia. *Pediatr Clin North Am.* 2007;54(5):672–689.[29]

are specific and developmentally based (e.g., fear of the dark, fear of separation, fear of death), whereas anxiety is a generalized feeling of uneasiness without a known source. Anxiety and depression may be comorbid conditions.

Anxiety in terminal illness is an expected reaction and should be assessed frequently. Toddlers and young children will generally have anxiety reactions that are an extension of the stress and anxiety levels of parents and other family members around them. These reactions may include irritability, clinginess, temper tantrums, and inconsolability. School-aged children and adolescents who can cognitively comprehend their illness and impending death may experience more adult-like symptoms, such as chronic apprehension, worry, difficulty concentrating, and sleep disturbance. Chaplains, child life workers, social workers, and psychologists are helpful in assessing children's fears, worries, and dreams. Children and adolescents under stress may regress behaviorally and emotionally; therefore, healthcare professionals should be alert to changes in the child's coping or personality.

Depression

Risk factors for depression in chronically ill children include frequent disruptions in important relationships, uncontrolled pain, and multiple physical disabilities.[31] Existential factors related to impending death, concern for parents and other family members, and a personal or family history of pre-existing psychological problems can also increase the risk for depression in chronically ill children. Suicidal thoughts are not common in terminally ill children and adolescents, but healthcare providers should be alert to comments about wishing to die and seek social workers, child life therapists, or psychologists to assist in further assessment and management.

Assessment of depressive symptoms must account for the child's developmental level. Psychologists, clinical social workers, and child life therapists have expertise in assisting children with life-threatening illnesses and should be consulted early in the trajectory to reduce psychological distress. Somatic complaints, such as lack of appetite, insomnia, agitation, and loss of energy, may be the result of disease and cannot be considered hallmark signs of depression. More appropriate signs would include a persistent sad face and demeanor, tearfulness, irritability, and withdrawal from previously enjoyed activities and relationships. Siblings may exhibit persistent and significant decrease in school performance, hypersomnolence, changes in appetite or weight, and nonspecific complaints of not feeling well. Parents should be assessed for depressed appearance, fearfulness, withdrawal, a sense of punishment, and mood that cannot be improved with good news. Referrals for further evaluation should be made as needed.[4]

Pharmacologic management of anxiety and depression should be considered if symptoms of anxiety and depression are debilitating. Consultation with psychiatric specialists for further evaluation and choice of agents is appropriate to assist with assessment and medication recommendations. Generally, management of anxiety and depression related to terminal illness in children involves nonpharmacologic interventions aimed at addressing the underlying issues. Both unconditional acceptance of the child's feelings and reassurance are powerful anxiety and depression interventions. Facilitating open communication between children and their parents may also be helpful.

Neurologic Symptoms

Restlessness and Agitation

Restlessness is a state of hyperarousal, not being able to rest or remain in a relaxed position. Agitation in children may present as irritability, combativeness, or refusal of attention or participation. Restlessness and agitation in children with advanced disease can be caused by a variety of physical and psychological causes (Box 2.7).

Assessment should include observing for frequent position changes, twitching, inability to concentrate on activities, inconsolability, disturbed sleep-wake cycles, and moaning. Spiritual distress, disturbing dreams

Box 2.7 Causes of Agitation and Restlessness in Children

Disease- and Treatment-Related Causes

Uncontrolled pain or other symptoms
Metabolic disturbances
Infections
Hypoxemia
Constipation
Sleep disturbance

Emotional Causes

Depression and anxiety
Fear
Change in family routine
Reaction to stress of other family members
Withholding of open information or open discussion with child

or nightmares, fears, and comorbid anxiety or depression should also be assessed. Treatment for agitation and restlessness should use both age-appropriate pharmacologic and nonpharmacologic techniques (Table 2.4). Sedation is generally indicated when distress cannot be controlled by any other means, because of either limited timeframe or risk for excessive morbidity. Healthcare professionals must determine what are truly uncontrollable pain or symptoms versus undertreated pain or symptoms. Before sedation, it is important that all efforts have been made to control pain and symptoms. The goal of palliative sedation is to relieve the child's obvious suffering by adding medications to induce sleep; it is not intended to hasten death.

Presenting a sedation option to a child and family requires a caring, open relationship between the treating healthcare professionals and the family. If the child and family are opposed to sedation, they should be reassured that all efforts to relieve distress will continue. If the child and family choose sedation, there are a number of pharmacologic agents available. Consultation with a hospice physician would be appropriate to determine the clinical appropriateness and best agents to use.

Seizures

The risk for seizures in advanced and terminal disease is related to the nature of the underlying disease.[33] Children with congenital malformations of the brain such as lissencephaly and congenital hydrocephaly, as well as other neurodegenerative diseases, often have seizures. Children with malignancies of the central nervous system may experience seizures, as an initial presentation of their illness or during disease progression. Children with advanced illnesses may also have seizure activity, as a result of metabolic abnormalities, hypoxia, and neurotoxicity from medications. Seizure activity in children can present in a number of ways (Box 2.8). No matter what the cause, uncontrolled seizure is often one of the most

Table 2.4 Management of Agitation and Restlessness

Intervention	Dose	Comments
Pharmacologic Management		
Lorazepam	0.03–0.1 mg IV/PO q4–6h, may titrate to max 2 mg/dose	Indicated for generalized anxiety
		May increase sedation in combination with opioids
		May use in infants and young children
Midazolam	0.025–0.05 mg/kg/dose IV/SC	Titrate to effect
	0.3–1 mg/kg (max 20 mg) PR	Indicated for myoclonus related to prolonged opioid use, mild sedation
		Short-acting, quickly reversed if overly sedated
Haloperidol	0.05–0.15 mg/kg/day PO, IV, SC divided 2–3 times per day	Indicated for agitation not responsive to benzodiazepines
		Monitor for extrapyramidal symptoms; treat with diphenhydramine as needed
Nonpharmacologic Management		
Maximize pain and other symptom assessment and management		
Decrease environmental stress or stimulation		
Encourage open communication between child and family		
Provide relaxation and guided imagery		
Provide favorite books, videos, or music		
Encourage cuddling or holding by parents and other significant family members		

From Wusthoff CJ, Shellhaas RA, Licht DJ. Management of common neurologic symptoms in pediatric palliative care: seizures, agitation, and spasticity. *Pediatr Clin North Am.* 2007;54(5):709–733.[32]

distressing symptoms for parents. If a child has any risk for seizure activity at the end of life, emergency medications such as diazepam suppositories should be available in the home. Management involves correcting the underlying cause when possible and adding appropriate prophylactic pharmacologic agents such as phenobarbital, clonazepam, or lorazepam (Table 2.5).

Box 2.8 Seizure Patterns in Children

Infants and Neonates

Deviation of eyes
Pedaling or stepping movements of legs
Rowing movements of arms
Eye blinking or fluttering
Sucking or smacking lips
Drooling
Apnea
Tonic-clonic movements

Older Children

Staring spells and deviated gaze
Unilateral or bilateral twitching, tremors
Generalized tonic-clonic movements

Respiratory Symptoms

Dyspnea

The experience of dyspnea is one of the most common nonpain symptoms reported by children and parents.[35-37] Dyspnea is the unpleasant sensation of breathlessness and can be particularly frightening for children. Diseases of childhood most associated with dyspnea include cystic fibrosis and other interstitial lung diseases, muscular dystrophy, spinal muscular atrophy, end-stage organ failure, and metastatic cancer. In each of these diseases, there can be a number of underlying causes (Box 2.9) that may be amenable to treatment.

The sensation of dyspnea is a subjective experience. Assessment should include effect on the child's functional status, factors that worsen or improve dyspnea, lung sounds, presence of pain with breathing, and oxygenation status. Extent of disease, respiratory rate, and oxygenation status may not always correlate with the degree of breathlessness experienced; therefore, patient report is the best indicator of the degree of distress. There is no validated tool to measure dyspnea. Using a rating similar to a pain scale measures distress and intervention response.

Early in the terminal process, respiratory discomfort interventions are aimed at improving respiratory effort. Antibiotics, oxygen, chemotherapy, or radiation to decrease tumor burden and noninvasive ventilation for children with muscular degenerative disease may be appropriate to treat the underlying cause. As the child becomes increasingly debilitated, the focus shifts to alleviating anxiety associated with respiratory changes and shortness of breath. There are a number of pharmacologic choices for managing respiratory symptoms (Table 2.6). Opioids are the treatment of choice for managing dyspnea, as well as for treating a persistent cough. Anticholinergic medications minimize secretions. Bronchodilators promote increased air exchange in the lungs and can be helpful alone or in conjunction with opioids. Anxiolytic drugs can help reduce anxiety related to shortness of breath and improve

Table 2.5 Management of Seizures at End of Life

Intervention	Dose	Comments
Phenobarbital	*Loading dose:* children 10–20 mg/kg IV, may titrate by 5 mg/kg increments q15–30 min until seizure controlled or to max of 40 mg/kg per dose	Generalized tonic-clonic seizures
	Maintenance dose: infants/children 5-8 mg/kg/day in 1–2 divided doses. Therapeutic serum levels 1–50 µg/mL	Status epilepticus
Carbamazepine	<6 y initial: 5 mg/kg/day PO, titrate based on serum levels q5–7 d to dose of 10 mg/day, then 20 mg/kg/day if necessary, give in 2–4 divided doses	Partial or complete seizures, generalized tonic-clonic, mixed seizure patterns
	6–12 y initial: 100 mg/day or 10 mg/kg/day PO in 2 divided doses, increase by 200 mg/day in weekly intervals until therapeutic serum levels reached	
	>12 y to adult, *initial*: 200 mg PO bid, increase by 200 mg/day in weekly intervals until therapeutic serum levels reached	
Phenytoin	*Loading dose:* infants/children 15–20 mg/kg IV	Generalized tonic-clonic seizures
	Maintenance dose: 6 mo to 3 y: 8–10 mg/kg/day in divided doses; 4 y–6 y: 7.5–9 mg/kg/day in divided doses; 7 y–9 y: 7–8 mg/kg/day in divided doses; 10 y–16 y: 6–7 mg/kg/day in divided doses	Status epilepticus
	Therapeutic levels: 8–15 µg/mL for neonates, 10–20 µg/mL for children	
Diazepam	2–5 y: 0.5 mg/kg PR 6–11 y: 0.3 mg/kg PR >11 y: 0.2 mg/kg PR May repeat 0.25 mg/kg in 10 min PRN	Status epilepticus

Adapted from Faulkner KW, Thayer PB, Coulter DL. Neurological and neuromuscular symptoms. In: Goldman A, Hain R, Liben S, eds. *Oxford Textbook of Palliative Care for Children.* London and New York: Oxford University Press; 2006:409-437.[34]

respiratory comfort.[35] It is important to determine, with the child and family, the level of intervention that is consistent with their perceptions of the child's suffering and quality of life.

Mechanical Ventilation in Pediatric Palliative Care

The use of long-term mechanical ventilation has increased significantly for children with chronic respiratory failure due to neuromuscular diseases and central nervous system malformations.[39-41] Approximately half of these patients had long-term ventilation initiated during a respiratory crisis,[42-44] putting families in the position to decide to let their child die or proceed with

Box 2.9 Causes of Dyspnea

Physiologic Causes

Tumor infiltration and compression

Aspiration

Pleural effusion, pulmonary edema, pneumothorax

Pneumonia

Thick secretions and mucous plugs

Bronchospasm

Impaired diaphragmatic excursion due to ascites, large abdominal tumors

Congestive heart failure

Respiratory muscle weakness due to progressive neurodegenerative disease

Metabolic disturbances

Psychological Causes

Anxiety

Panic disorder

mechanical ventilation.[45] Children with complex chronic conditions are more likely to require invasive ventilation by tracheostomy, have lower levels of cognitive capacity, experience poorer quality of life and functional status, and experience death as the outcome of mechanical ventilation.[40,42,46-48]

Terminal Respirations

In the final days to hours of life, respiratory patterns often change, initially becoming more rapid and shallow, then progressing to deep, slow respirations with periods of apnea, know as Cheyne-Stokes breathing.[37] As the body weakens, pooling of secretions in the throat can lead to noisy respirations, sometimes referred to as "death rattle." Often at this point, children are somnolent most of the time and do not report distress. These symptoms, however, are particularly agonizing for parents and other family members. Assessment should include changes in heart and respiratory rate, observing for distress, stridor, wheezing, and rales and rhonchi. Management should focus on managing family distress by explaining the nature of the dying process, reassuring the family that the child is not suffering, administering appropriate anticholinergic medications to decrease secretions, and decreasing or discontinuing any fluids or enteral feedings that may exacerbate the development of secretions or fluid overload.

Summary

Suffering from uncontrolled symptoms can be prevented by knowledge of the child's underlying disease process, thorough assessment of the child and family for sources of suffering, advocacy for child and family needs, and use of an interdisciplinary approach to management that includes appropriate pharmacologic and nonpharmacologic interventions.

Table 2.6 Management of Respiratory Symptoms

Agent	Dose	Comments
Morphine	0.1–0.2 mg/kg/dose IV/ SC	Indicated for dyspnea, cough
	0.2–0.5 mg/kg/dose PO	May need to titrate to comfort
Hydromorphone	15 µg/kg IV q4–6h	
	0.03–0.08 mg/kg/dose PO q4–6h	
Glycopyrrolate	40–100 mg/kg/dose PO 3–4 times/ day	Indicated for secretions, congestion
	4–10 µg/kg/dose IV/SC q3–4h	May give in conjunction with hyoscyamine
Hyoscyamine	Infant drops (<2 y)	
	• 2.3 kg: 3 gtts q4h; max: 18 gtt/day	
	• 3.4 kg: 4 gtt q4h; 24 gtt/day	
	• 5 kg: 5 gtt q4h; max: 30 gtt/day	
	• 7 kg: 6 gtt q4h; max: 36 gtt/day	
	• 10 kg: 8 gtt q4h; 48 gtt/day	
	• 15 kg: 10 gtt q4h; 66 gtt/day	
	2–12 y: 0.0625–0.125 mg PO q4h; max: 0.75 mg/day	
	>12 y: 0.125–0.25 mg PO q4h; max: 1.5 mg/day	
Hydromet (solution combination of hydrocodone and homatropine)	0.6 mg/kg/day divided 3–4 doses/ day	
Albuterol	Oral: 2–6 y: 0.1–0.2 mg/kg/ dose tid; max: 4 mg tid	Indicated for wheezing, pulmonary congestion
	6–12 y: 2 mg/dose 3–4 times/day; max: 24 mg/ day	Side effects include increased heart rate, anxiety
	>12 y: 2–4 mg/dose 3–4 times/day; max: 8 mg qid	
	Nebulized: 0.01–0.5 mL/kg of 0.5% solution q4–6h	

Adapted from Lieben S, Hain R, Goldman A. Respiratory symptoms. In: Goldman A, Hain R, Liben S, eds. *Oxford Textbook of Palliative Care for Children.* London and New York: Oxford University Press; 2006:438-447.[38]

References

1. Kogan MD, Strickland BB, Newacheck PW. Building systems of care: findings from the National Survey of Children With Special Health Care Needs. *Pediatrics.* 2009;124(Suppl 4):S333-336.

2. Rehm RS. Nursing's contribution to research about parenting children with complex chronic conditions: an integrative review, 2002 to 2012. *Nurs Outlook.* 2013;61(5):266-290.

3. Cohen E, Berry JG, Camacho X, et al. Patterns and costs of health care use of children with medical complexity. *Pediatrics.* 2012;130(6):e1463-e1470.

4. Schwab A, Rusconi-Serpa S, Schechter DS. Psychodynamic approaches to medically ill children and their traumatically stressed parents. *Child Adolesc Psychiatr Clin N Am.* 2013;22(1):119-139.

5. Jantien Vrijmoet-Wiersma CM, van Klink JM, Kolk AM, et al. Assessment of parental psychological stress in pediatric cancer: a review. *J Pediatr Psychol.* 2008;33(7):694-706.

6. Alvesson HM, Lindelow M, Khanthaphat B, Laflamme L. Coping with uncertainty during healthcare-seeking in Lao PDR. *BMC Int Health Hum Rights.* 2013;13(1):28.

7. Barrera M, Granek L, Shaheed J, et al. The tenacity and tenuousness of hope: parental experiences of hope when their child has a poor cancer prognosis. *Cancer Nurs.* 2013;36(5):408-416.

8. Tong A, Lowe A, Sainsbury P, Craig JC. Experiences of parents who have children with chronic kidney disease: a systematic review of qualitative studies. *Pediatrics.* 2008;121(2):349-360.

9. Granek L, Barrera M, Shaheed J, et al. Trajectory of parental hope when a child has difficult-to-treat cancer: a prospective qualitative study. *Psychooncology.* 2013;22(11):2436-2444.

10. Lerret SM, Weiss ME. How ready are they? Parents of pediatric solid organ transplant recipients and the transition from hospital to home following transplant. *Pediatr Transplant.* 2011;15(6):606-616.

11. Stewart JL, Pyke-Grimm KA, Kelly KP. Making the right decision for my child with cancer: the parental imperative. *Cancer Nurs.* 2012;35(6):419-428.

12. Tong A, Lowe A, Sainsbury P, Craig JC. Parental perspectives on caring for a child with chronic kidney disease: an in-depth interview study. *Child Care Health Dev.* 2010;36(4):549-557.

13. Malcolm C, Gibson F, Adams S, et al. A relational understanding of sibling experiences of children with rare life-limiting conditions: findings from a qualitative study. *J Child Health Care.* 2014;18(3):230-240.

14. Wolfe J, Grier HE, Klar N, et al. Symptoms and suffering at the end of life in children with cancer. *N Engl J Med.* 2000;342(5):326-333.

15. Whitsett SF, Gudmundsdottir M, Davies B, et al. Chemotherapy-related fatigue in childhood cancer: correlates, consequences, and coping strategies. *J Pediatr Oncol Nurs.* 2008;25(2):86-96.

16. Ullrich CK, Mayer OH. Assessment and management of fatigue and dyspnea in pediatric palliative care. *Pediatr Clin North Am.* 2007;54(5):735-756.

17. Karwacki MW. Gastrointestinal symptoms. In: Goldman A, Hain R, Liben S, eds. *Oxford Textbook of Palliative Care for Children.* London and New York: Oxford University Press; 2006:342-372.

18. Dupuis LL, Boodhan S, Holdsworth M, et al. Guideline for the prevention of acute nausea and vomiting due to antineoplastic medication in pediatric cancer patients. *Pediatr Blood Cancer*. 2013;60(7):1073-1082.

19. Phillips RS, Gopaul S, Gison F, et al. Antiemetic medication for prevention and treatment of chemotherapy induced nausea and vomiting in childhood. *Cochrane Database Syst Rev*. 2010(9):CD007786.

20. Chen S, Jarboe MD, Teitelbaum DH. Effectiveness of a transluminal endoscopic fundoplication for the treatment of pediatric gastroesophageal reflux disease. *Pediatr Surg Int*. 2012;28(3):229-234.

21. Mahant S, Friedman JN, Connolly B, et al. Tube feeding and quality of life in children with severe neurological impairment. *Arch Dis Child*. 2009;94(9):668-673.

22. Marchand, V. Nutrition in neurologically impaired children. *Paediatr Child Health*. 2009;14(6):395-401.

23. Riley A, Vadeboncoeur C. Nutritional differences in neurologically impaired children. *Paediatr Child Health*. 2012;17(9):e98-e101.

24. Morgan AT, Dodrill P, Ward EC. Interventions for oropharyngeal dysphagia in children with neurological impairment. *Cochrane Database Syst Rev*. 2012;10:CD009456.

25. Zaidi T, Sudall C, Kauffmann L, et al. Physical outcome and quality of life after total esophagogastric dissociation in children with severe neurodisability and gastroesophageal reflux, from the caregiver's perspective. *J Pediatr Surg*. 2010;45(9):1772-1776.

26. Srivastava R, Downey EC, O'Gorman M, et al. Impact of fundoplication versus gastrojejunal feeding tubes on mortality and in preventing aspiration pneumonia in young children with neurologic impairment who have gastroesophageal reflux disease. *Pediatrics*. 2009;123(1):338-345.

27. Mak RH, Cheung WW, Zhan JY, et al. Cachexia and protein-energy wasting in children with chronic kidney disease. *Pediatr Nephrol*. 2012;27(2):173-181.

28. Rodgers CC, Hooke MC, Hockenberry MJ. Symptom clusters in children. *Curr Opin Support Palliat Care*. 2013;7(1):67-72.

29. Santucci G, Mack JW. Common gastrointestinal symptoms in pediatric care: nausea, vomiting, constipation, anorexia, cachexia. *Pediatr Clin North Am*. 2007;54(5):672-689.

30. Tsai, E. Withholding and withdrawing artificial nutrition and hydration. *Paediatr Child Health*. 2011;16(4):241-244.

31. Muriel AC, McCulloch R, Hammel JF. Depression, anxiety, and delirium. In: Goldman A, Hain R, Liben S, eds. *Oxford Textbook of Palliative Care for Children*. London and New York: Oxford University Press; 2012:309-318.

32. Wusthoff CJ, Shellhaas RA, Licht DJ. Management of common neurologic symptoms in pediatric palliative care: Seizures, agitation, and spasticity. *Pediatr Clin North Am*. 2007;54(5):709-733.

33. Hauer JM, Faulkner KW. Neurological and neuromuscular conditions and symptoms. In: Goldman A, Hain R, Liben S, eds. *Oxford Textbook of Palliative Care for Children*. London and New York: Oxford University Press; 2012:295-308.

34. Faulkner KW, Thayer PB, Coulter DL. Neurological and neuromuscular symptoms. In: Goldman A, Hain R, Liben S, eds. *Oxford Textbook of Palliative Care for Children*. London and New York: Oxford University Press; 2006:409-437.

35. Robinson WM. Palliation of dyspnea in pediatrics. *Chron Respir Dis.* 2012;9(4):251-256.

36. Schindera C, Tomlinson D, Bartels U, et al. Predictors of symptoms and site of death in pediatric palliative patients with cancer at end of life. *Am J Hosp Palliat Care.* 2014;31(5):548-552.

37. Brook L, Twig E, Venables A, Shaw, C. Respiratory symptoms. In: Goldman A, Hain R, Liben S, eds. *Oxford Textbook of Palliative Care for Children.* London and New York: Oxford University Press; 2012:319-327.

38. Lieben S, Hain R, Goldman A. Respiratory symptoms. In: Goldman A, Hain R, Liben S, eds. *Oxford Textbook of Palliative Care for Children.* London and New York: Oxford University Press; 2006:438-447.

39. Divo MJ, Murray S, Cortopassi F, Celli BR. Prolonged mechanical ventilation in massachusetts: the 2006 prevalence survey. *Respir Care.* 2010; 55(12);1693-1698.

40. Edwards JD, Kun SS, Keens TG. Outcomes and causes of death in children on home mechanical ventilation via tracheostomy: an institutional and literature review. *J Pediatr.* 2010;157(6):955-959, e952.

41. Goodwin S, Smith H, Langton Hewer S, et al. Increasing prevalence of domiciliary ventilation: changes in service demand and provision in the South West of the UK. *Eur J Pediatr.* 2011;170(9):1187-1192.

42. Edwards JD, Kun SS, Graham RJ, Keens TG. End-of-Life discussions and advance care planning for children on long-term assisted ventilation with life-limiting conditions. *J Palliat Care.* 2012;(1):21-27.

43. Ottonello G, Ferrari I, Pirroddi IM, et al. Home mechanical ventilation in children: retrospective survey of a pediatric population. *Pediatr Int.* 2007;49(6):801-805.

44. Wallis C, Paton JY, Beaton S, Jardine E. Children on long-term ventilatory support: 10 years of progress. *Arch Dis Child.* 2011;96(11):998-1002.

45. Carnevale FA, Alexander E, Davis M, et al. Daily living with distress and enrichment: the moral experience of families with ventilator-assisted children at home. *Pediatrics.* 2006;117(1):e48-e60.

46. Dybwik K, Nielsen EW, Brinchmann BS. Ethical challenges in home mechanical ventilation: a secondary analysis. *Nurs Ethics.* 2012;19(2):233-244.

47. Kun SS, Edwards JD, Ward SL, Keens TG. Hospital readmissions for newly discharged pediatric home mechanical ventilation patients. *Pediatr Pulmonol.* 2012;47(4):409-414.

48. Reiter K, Pernath N, Pagel P, et al. Risk factors for morbidity and mortality in pediatric home mechanical ventilation. *Clin Pediatr* (Phila). 2011;50(3):237-243.

Chapter 3

Pediatric Pain

Knowing the Child Before You

Mary Layman Goldstein and Dana Kramer

Expert pain management is a crucial part of pediatric palliative care. It is possible for children of all ages to feel and express pain. A child's ability to communicate about pain is influenced by age and cognitive level,[1] but even a preverbal child can communicate about pain. To effectively manage the pain of an individual child, the nurse first must be aware of the possibility of pain, sensitively observe the child, and use developmentally appropriate, objective assessments. Developmental factors (physical, emotional, and cognitive) play an important role in both pediatric pain assessment and pain management.

Definitions of Pain and Other Relevant Terms

Pain has been described as "an unpleasant emotional experience associated with actual or potential tissue damage or described in terms of such damage."[2] Another definition, penned by Margo McCaffery, RN, in 1968, highlights the subjective nature of pain. According to McCaffery, pain is "whatever the experiencing person says it is, experienced whenever they say they are experiencing it."[3]

Nociception is "the perception by the nerves of injurious influences or painful stimuli."[2] This term is frequently used in discussions of pain in the neonate because of the challenges in evaluating the newborn's (preterm up to age 1 month) perception of pain. See Table 3.1 for useful questions in evaluating a child with pain.

Prevalence of Pain in Children

Clinicians working with children in the general pediatric area will encounter pain in children who are undergoing immunizations and procedures and in those who have pharyngitis, oral viral infection, otitis media, urinary tract infection, headache, or traumatic injury. Pain continues to be present in children with cancer at the end of life. Conditions such as meningitis and necrotizing colitis can cause pain in children. Children who experience chronic

Table 3.1 Useful Questions in Evaluating a Child With Pain

Question	Clinical Implications of Answers
What is the chronologic age of the child?	Age-related physiologic development affects pharmacokinetic and pharmacodynamic effects of medications.
	In the neonate, normal neuroanatomic and neurobiologic developmental processes occur and allow for transmission of painful stimuli.
What is the developmental stage of the child?	Developmental age helps determine:
• Neonate • Infant • Toddler • Preschooler or young child • School-aged child • Adolescent	• How a child might express his or her pain • Which assessment tools may be useful • What cognitive-behavioral techniques might be considered
What type of pain does the child have?	The particular situation can guide the clinician to a developmentally appropriate assessment tool and a situation-specific pain management plan that includes both pharmacologic and nonpharmacologic interventions.
• Acute pain • Chronic pain • Procedural pain	
Does the child have a chronic illness?	Certain painful conditions have disease-specific, validated pain assessment tools. For example, the Douleur Enfant Gustave Roussy (DEGR) scale is available to assess prolonged pain in 2- to 6-year-olds with cancer[a]
Is the child neurologically impaired?	Cognitively impaired children may process information and communicate distress differently from normally developed children[b]
	Besides knowing the science, and the individual child, it may help to know other children with similar conditions[b]
	New pain assessment tools for children with intellectual disabilities are being validated to look at generic, procedural, and surgical pain[b]
Do the child and parents speak the same language as healthcare providers?	Find ways of obtaining translators.
	Some pain assessment tools are available in translated versions[c]
	It may be worth having pain assessment tools translated into languages common to certain practice settings.
What is the underlying cause of the pain?	If the underlying cause is treatable, the pain may be reduced or eliminated.

(continued)

Table 3.1 (Continued)

Question	Clinical Implications of Answers
What is the child's weight in kilograms?	Dosage of analgesics is expressed in milligrams or micrograms per kilogram.
	For some medications, the starting dose depends on the child's being larger or smaller than a set weight.
Is the oral route of drug administration used whenever possible?	Besides being a cheaper and less invasive route (with less potential for pain and infection), the oral route in children provides more reliable absorption.
Are there any obvious, outstanding barriers that may be playing a role in the child's pain assessment and management?	Some barriers can be directly and quickly addressed with minimal effect and maximal positive impact.
Have nonpharmacologic pain interventions been considered?	Nonpharmacologic pain interventions based on the etiology of a child's pain can improve the comprehensiveness and effectiveness of a pain management plan.

ᵃ Adapted from Gauvain-Piquard et al.[4]
ᵇ Adapted from Knegt et al.[5]
ᶜ Adapted from Silva &Thuler.[6]

diseases such as cancer, HIV infection, sickle cell disease (SCD), hemophilia, juvenile chronic arthritis, and cystic fibrosis also will have pain.

Etiology of Pain in Children

Neuropathic Pain

Neuropathic pain is less common in children than in adults. Many of the neuropathic pain syndromes seen in adults are not diagnosed as frequently in children. Children may experience neuropathic pain from migraine headaches, scar neuromas after surgery, phantom limb pain after amputations for trauma, tumors, meningococcemia, autoimmune and degenerative neuropathies, and complex regional pain syndromes (reported in preteen and teenage girls).[1] Neuropathic pain is also common in pediatric cancer patients for a number of reasons, discussed in more detail later.

Burns

Burns, which can sometimes be life threatening, are thermal injuries caused by hot liquids, flames, and electricity; they are among the most common causes of injury to children and are associated with pain. This injury, which destroys the skin, can have significant morbidity and mortality, depending on the extent of the burn. Intact skin is necessary for protection against bacterial infection, fluid and electrolyte balance, and thermoregulation. Treatment of severe burns is associated with significant pain. Undertreatment of this pain can make it difficult for the child to cooperate with burn treatment.

Cancer

The World Health Organization stated that 70% of children with cancer will experience severe pain during their illness.[7] The types of pain in children with cancer, whether caused by procedures, the disease or tumor, or anticancer treatment, have been well described for many years.[8,9] This pain can be acute or chronic. Children with chronic cancer-related pain frequently experience breakthrough pain.[1]

All children with cancer are at risk for procedural pain. Most procedure-related pain involves needle puncture. This procedure may be necessary for obtaining blood supplies, accessing implanted venous devices, administering intravenous chemotherapeutics, or giving intramuscular or subcutaneous medications. Lumbar punctures (using a spinal needle) and bone marrow aspiration (involving insertion of a large needle into the posterior superior iliac spine) are variations of needle puncture. Some children develop pro-longed post–lumbar puncture headaches.[10] Despite significant efforts to avoid needlesticks in the pediatric population, sometimes a needle puncture is necessary and cannot be avoided. Removal of tunneled central venous catheters or implanted ports also causes procedural pain and must be addressed by clinicians caring for children undergoing this procedure.[8]

For some children, it is the experience of tumor-related pain that leads their parents to seek medical attention and eventual diagnosis. This pain can be nociceptive or neuropathic. Nociceptive pain can be somatic, caused by tumor involvement with bone or soft tissue, or visceral, caused by tumor infiltration, compression, or distention of abdominal or thoracic viscera. Neuropathic pain can be caused by tumor involvement (i.e., compression or infiltration) with the peripheral or central nervous system.

Most children who receive a diagnosis of cancer, no matter what the stage, will receive some sort of anticancer treatment. Frequently, this treatment causes some sort of pain, either acute or chronic. Surgery leads to acute, postoperative pain. Removal of limbs may lead to the development of phantom limb sensations and pain. This experience is thought to decrease over time in children. Radiation therapy may lead to an acute dermatitis or pain. Children undergoing chemotherapy are at risk acutely for mucositis pain and gastritis from repeated vomiting (if nausea and vomiting are not successfully controlled)[8] and chronically for neuropathic pain from certain chemotherapies. Children who have been treated with high doses of steroids are at risk for development of avascular necrosis, a disabling condition that eventually causes the affected bone to collapse. Some chemotherapy agents, such as vincristine, asparaginase, and cyclophosphamide, can cause pain or painful conditions, such as peripheral neuropathy, constipation, hemorrhagic cystitis, or pancreatitis. Complications of intravenous chemotherapy administration may lead to pain from irritation, infiltration, extravasation, tissue necrosis (if vesicants are used), or the development of thrombophlebitis. Children receiving intrathecal chemotherapy may develop arachnoiditis or meningeal irritation, also painful conditions. The child who is immunocompromised, whether from chemotherapy or from disease, is at risk for infection and infection-related pain. Skin, perioral, and perirectal infections are common. Children seem to be at less risk for acute herpes zoster and its related pain.[1] Bone marrow transplantation may lead acutely to severe mucositis and potentially to chronic graft-versus-host disease, which may manifest as severe abdominal pain if it affects the gastrointestinal system.[8]

Medications used to prevent or modify side effects of primary disease treatment can have painful effects. Use of corticosteroids in disease treatment may lead to bone changes that cause pain.[11] Colony-stimulating factors may lead to medullary bone pain shortly after administration and before the onset of neutrophil recovery.

Human Immunodeficiency Virus Infection

Children with HIV infection may experience pain for a variety of reasons, including disease, treatment, and procedures. Some factors are quite similar to those associated with cancer-related pain, and some are unique to HIV disease.

Sickle Cell Disease

One of the most common genetic diseases in the United States, commonly affecting individuals of African, Middle Eastern, Mediterranean, and Indian descent, is highly associated with a variety of painful conditions. SCD is characterized by a predominance of hemoglobin S, which becomes sickle-shaped (as opposed to donut-shaped) after deoxygenation. It is this stiff, sickle-shaped red blood cell that becomes trapped in small blood vessels, leading to vasoocclusion, tissue ischemia, and even infarction.[1]

Some of the many painful states that are commonly associated with SCD include acute painful events, acute hand-foot syndrome, acute inflammation of joints, acute chest syndrome, splenic sequestration, intrahepatic sickling or hepatic sequestration, avascular necrosis of femur or humerus, and priapism. The reader is directed to the American Pain Society's *Guidelines for the Management of Acute and Chronic Pain in Sickle Cell Disease*[12(p3-7)] for a review of the clinical signs and symptoms of these and other common SCD pain states, their underlying causes, and special features or considerations.

Other Conditions Associated With Pain in Children

Other conditions children experience that may be associated with pain include cystic fibrosis, muscular dystrophy and other degenerative neurologic diseases, and severe dermatologic conditions. A recent study of children with hemiplegic cerebral palsy, identified from a population register, revealed that 33% had mild pain and 18% had moderate to severe pain.[13]

Physiology and Pathophysiology of Pain in Children

Those working with children need to be aware of the normal neuroanatomic and neurobiologic developmental processes that occur in neonates and allow for the development of transmission of painful stimuli (Table 3.2). In fact, there is strong evidence to suggest that neonates have increased sensitivity to pain because the inhibitory pain tracts are the last to develop.[14] It is possible to

Table 3.2 Pain-Related Developmental Milestones

Age	Development	Assessment and Management Implications
7 wk gestation	Pain receptors present[a]	
20 wk gestation	Full compliment of neurons in cerebral cortex[a]	
	Pain receptors spread to all cutaneous and mucosal surfaces[a]	
26 wk gestation	Can respond to tissue injury as demonstrated by "specific behavioral, autonomic, hormonal, and metabolic signs of stress and distress" (p. 1094) due to sufficient development of peripheral, spinal, and supraspinal afferent pain transmission pathways[a]	
30 wk gestation	Myelination usually complete[a]	
	Slower transmission of pain thought to be offset by decreased distance the impulse must travel[a]	
40 wk gestation	Descending, inhibitory pathways, which alter and modulate pain perception, present[a]	
Neonate (preterm through 1 mo)	**Acute pain responses:**	
	• Physiologic measures, such as increase in vital signs, are similar to those of older children and adults	• Challenging to differentiate symptoms of pain (a stressful situation) from other life-threatening situations such as hypoxemia[b]
	• Behavioral indicators include vocalizations (crying, whimpering, groaning), facial expression changes (grimaces, furrowed brow, quivering chin, tightly closed eyes, square open mouth), body movement and posture (thrashing, limb withdrawn, fist clenched, flaccidity), and other behavior changes (sleep-wake cycle, feeding, activity, irritability or listlessness)[a]	
		• Validated composite measures include the Neonatal Infant Pain Scale, or NIPS[c]; the CRIES postoperative pain tool[d] (C = crying; R = requires increased oxygen administration; I = increased vital signs; E = expression; S = sleeplessness), and the Premature Infant Pain Profile (PIPPS)[e]

(continued)

Table 3.2 (Continued)

Age	Development	Assessment and Management Implications
	• Chronic responses can include changes or disruptions in usual feeding, activity, and sleep-wake patterns	• One-dimensional pain assessment measure: Neonatal Facial Coding System[f]
		• Measures do not address neonates with chronic pain, those pharmacologically paralyzed for mechanical ventilation, or those with significant facial deformity[b]
	Physiologic developmental issues[i]:	
	• Increased water and volume of distribution for water-soluble medications	• Need for increased dosing interval or decreased rates of infusion for many medications[a]
	• Decreased fat and muscle	• Vulnerable to effects of decreased ventilatory reflexes[a]
	• Immature hepatic enzyme systems, leading to decreased metabolic clearances	
	• Decreased glomerular filtration rates, producing accumulation of renally excreted medications and active metabolites	
	• Many factors in respiratory function lead to increased risk for hypoventilation, atelectasis, or respiratory failure	
Infants (older than 1 mo)	**Acute pain responses:**	
	• Behavioral changes, physiologic responses, and facial responses of neonates exhibited[a]	• Examine infants older than 1 mo in parent's lap[g]
		• Children's Hospital of Eastern Ontario Pain Scale (CHEOPS)[h]
	• May cry loudly, thrash, arch, or exhibit body rigidity[a]	
	• Local reflex withdrawal of stimulated area in young infants[a]	
	• Deliberate withdrawal of affected area in older infants[a]	
	• Development of stranger anxiety after 7 mo[g]	
	Physiologic developmental issues[i]:	
	• Immature hepatic enzyme systems, leading to decreased metabolic clearances	• Need for increased dosing interval or decreased rates of infusion for many medications[a]
	• From birth to 7 mo, decreased glomerular filtration rates produce accumulation of renally excreted medications and active metabolites	• Vulnerable to effects of decreased ventilatory reflexes in response to opioids or sedatives[a]

(continued)

Table 3.2 (Continued)

Age	Development	Assessment and Management Implications
	• By 8 to 12 mo, renal blood flow, glomerular filtration, and tubular secretion increase to near adult values	
	• Many factors in respiratory function lead to increased risk for hypoventilation, atelectasis, or respiratory failure	
Toddlers	Behavioral changes (such as changes in eating, play-activity, and sleep-wake patterns) and physiologic responses as described in neonates[a]	Give toddler time to get used to you and build trust[g]
		Use play and minimized physical contact during physical assessment[g]
	May also cry intensely, be verbally aggressive, or withdraw from play or social interaction[a,g]	
		Language development varies, and it is best to use words for pain that are most familiar to a particular child[g]
	May have words for pain by 18 mo[h]	
	Stranger anxiety persists[g]	
	From age 2 to 6 y, children have a larger liver mass per kilogram of body weight, and this is thought to increase metabolic clearance of many medications	Often, it is beneficial to have parents present during assessment and procedures[i,j]
		By age 2 y, dosing intervals may be decreased or infusion rates increased because of increased metabolic clearance[a]
Preschooler (young child, age 3–6 y)	Behavioral changes (such as changes in eating, play-activity, and sleep-wake patterns) and physiologic responses as described in neonates[a]	Physical and emotional support by adults present, especially parents, may be comforting[j]
		Consider building on "magical thinking" abilities when initiating nonpharmacologic interventions[j]
	Developmentally able to give meaningful, concrete information about location and severity of pain[b,i]	
	Able to anticipate painful events/procedures[a]	Offer realistic choices if possible, and provide positive reinforcement[g]
	Behaviors may include clinging, lack of cooperation, attempts to push painful stimuli away before their application[a]	

(continued)

Table 3.2 (Continued)

Age	Development	Assessment and Management Implications
		By age 2 y, dosing intervals may be decreased or infusion rates increased because of increased metabolic clearance[a]
	"Magical thinking" (mixes facts and fiction)[j]	
	Pain may be viewed as a punishment or as a source of secondary gain[a]	
	From age 2 to 6 y, children have a larger liver mass per kilogram of body weight, and this is thought to increase metabolic clearance of many medications	
School-age child	Behavioral changes (such as changes in eating, play-activity, and sleep-wake patterns) and physiologic responses as described in neonates[a]	Child able to use more objective measures of pain, give more specific and detailed reports
		Able to use more cognitive coping methods, including educational interventions
	May exhibit rigid muscularity (gritted teeth, contracted limbs, stiff body, closed eyes, or wrinkled forehead)	
		Cultural beliefs may influence child's pain experience[a,k]
	May demonstrate more stalling behaviors to delay potentially painful experiences	
	Continued normal cognitive development influences ability to both report and learn information	
	May demonstrate influences of cultural group[k]	
Adolescent	Behavioral changes (such as changes in eating, play-activity, and sleep-wake patterns) and physiologic responses as described in neonates[a]	May deny pain in presence of peers
		May be influenced by cultural factors regarding interpretations and expressions of pain[a,k]
	May show more decreased motor activity in presence of pain	Parents remain advocate for child, but teenagers, if they so desire, need to be involved in decision-making[g]
		Validated multidimensional pain measurement tool available in English and Spanish for use in adolescents and children with different medical conditions: Adolescent Pediatric Pain Tool (APPT).[l]

(continued)

Table 3.2 (Continued)

Age	Development	Assessment and Management Implications
	Continued normal cognitive development	
	Increased influence of peers and cultural group[g,k]	
	Increased needs for privacy and independence[g]	
	Adolescent not legally independent (except in special cases) but needs to have a larger emerging role in his or her care[g]	

[a] Adapted from Berde & Setna.[16]
[b] Adapted from American Academy of Pediatrics & Canadian Pediatric Society.[15]
[c] Adapted from Lawrence et al.[17]
[d] Adapted from Krechel & Bildner.[18]
[e] Adapted from Stevens et al.[19]
[f] Adapted from Grunau & Craig.[20]
[g] Adapted from Levetown.[21]
[h] Adapted from McGrath et al.[22]
[i] Adapted from Cramton & Gruchala.[10]
[j] Adapted from Power et al.[23]
[k] Adapted from Davies et al.[24]
[l] Adapted from Jacob et al.[25]

assess the severity of pain and the effects of analgesics in neonates. Neonates who do not cry, move, or show other behavioral response to painful stimuli may still be experiencing pain. It has been shown that increased neonatal morbidity and mortality may result from prolonged or severe pain. In addition, neonates who experience pain may respond differently to pain later on (e.g., pain from inoculation or circumcision) than do those who have not experienced previous painful events.[15]

Assessment of Pain in Children

Assessment of pain in pediatrics involves a conversation between the clinician, the child, and the parents. The nurse must first learn who the child is to effectively treat the child's pain. To do this, nurses, evaluating pain in children of all ages, must be aware of potential barriers and influencing factors that may play a role in accurate, developmentally appropriate assessment. Table 3.3 reviews these barriers in detail.

Poor communication between the pediatric patient, family, and healthcare team increases the likelihood of suboptimal pain assessment and management. Factors that may interfere with assessment include language or cultural differences between, child, family, and clinicians; the presence of chronic health conditions, developmental disabilities, or cognitive, sensory, or motor impairments; and severe emotional disturbance.[29]

Table 3.3 Pediatric-Specific Barriers to Pain Control

Issue	Barrier/Misconception
Inadequate assessment	*Misconception:* Infants and children do not feel pain in the same way as adults do.[a]
	Misconception: Children are unable to provide useful, accurate information about the location and severity of their pain.[a]
	Lack of knowledge about how to assess pediatric pain[b]
	Challenge of pain assessment in preverbal or noncommunicating children
	Choosing the correct population-specific tool
Inadequate analgesics ordered or administered	Need for comprehensive assessment with pain etiology and contributing or modifying factors identified
	Need to select most appropriate medications, doses, dosing intervals, and route of administration for situation[c]
	Nurses' or parents' failure to administer the complete dose ordered or as frequently as ordered
	Prescriber's reluctance to send children home with the effective opioids that the child received while hospitalized[d]
Incorrect attitudes or misconceptions by patients, families, or healthcare providers about pain and its management	*Misconception:* Pain control in children is too difficult or time-consuming.[a]
	Lack of knowledge or incorrect knowledge of pharmacokinetics and pharmacodynamics of analgesics, especially opioids[b]
	Lack of knowledge of the consequences of unrelieved pain[b]
	Misconception: Children can tolerate pain better than adults (this can lead to heightened pain and anxiety about pain control).[b]
	Fear of opioid-related side effects and lack of knowledge about how to manage them can also prevent appropriate use of opioids in children.[b]
Systems-related issues	Need for systematic reevaluation and reassessment of pain management plan's effectiveness[b]
	No systematic, evidenced-based approach to pain management despite rigorous approach to other aspects of a child's care, including disease diagnosis and treatment
	Lack of appropriate use of nondrug therapies to complement or supplement the pharmacologic interventions[b]

(continued)

Table 3.3 (Continued)	
Issue	**Barrier/Misconception**
	Lack of knowledge by healthcare professionals of simple and practical physical, cognitive, or behavioral strategies that can give children and their families more control and less anxiety about pain management
	Lack of clear delineation of who is responsible for a particular child's pain control, leading to gaps in management[b]

[a] Adapted from Levine D et al. [26]
[b] Adapted from McGrath & Brown.[27]
[c] Adapted from World Health Organization.[1]
[d] Adapted from Field & Behrman.[28]

In learning who an individual child is, the nurse must interview the child as well as the parents. Choosing the appropriate pain assessment tool for a pediatric patient can be challenging. First, consider the developmental level and age of the child. Next, consider the type of pain, the context or specific illness, before selecting a tool. Attempts at measurement of pain include physiologic measures, behavioral observations, composite measures, and self-report.

Self-report, the gold standard in pain assessment, can be obtained from some children as young as age 3 years and generally by 6 years. Most pediatric self-report tools are not multidimensional and measure only pain intensity.[1] To adequately report detailed ratings of pain intensity, a child, usually of school age or older, must understand the concepts of sequence and numbering.

Assessment of pain begins with screening. Screening for pain can occur routinely from the time a child enters a healthcare system through simple documentation tools. Hospitalized children may be screened more than once a day for any changes in pain or for unsatisfactory pain control. The QUESTT approach to pediatric pain assessment is a simple guideline for proactive pain management and reevaluation,[30] as follows:

Question the child and parent.
Use pain-rating scales appropriate to developmental stage of the child and to the situation at hand.
Evaluate behavioral and physiologic changes.
Secure parents' involvement.
Take the cause of pain into account.
Take action and evaluate results.

In every practice setting, a child with pain needs regular reassessment to improve or maintain safe and effective management of pain.

Management

Pharmacologic Management

Nurses caring for children with pain must be aware of physiologic variations among different age groups that may affect analgesic action. Many pediatric analgesic studies in children are limited because they include a wide age range. This makes it challenging to distinguish between the effects of developmentally dependent physiologic processes that play a role in analgesia. Consider the potential for pathophysiologic differences in pediatric patients, including those in the body compartments, hepatic enzyme systems, plasma protein binding, renal filtration and excretion of medications and their metabolites, metabolic rate, oxygen consumption, and respiratory function. Table 3.2 presents some of these developmental physiologic changes and their clinical implications. Tables 3.4, 3.5, 3.6, 3.7, and 3.8 suggest starting doses for opioids and nonopioids that reflect these developmental aspects of pediatric pharmacology.

There are three main groups of medications used to treat pain in children: (1) nonopioids (e.g., acetaminophen, nonsteroidal antiinflammatory drugs [NSAIDs]), (2) opioids, and (3) adjuvant analgesics. Use of these medications depends on the severity and cause of pain in an individual child. The nonopioids and opioids are most helpful in the treatment of nociceptive pain, and adjuvant analgesics work best for specific neuropathic pain.

Use of Nonopioids in Children

Nonopioids (acetaminophen, NSAIDs, and aspirin) have a ceiling effect and cannot be safely titrated beyond the dose per weight given at drug-specific intervals. Pediatric dosage guidelines for commonly used nonopioid analgesics can be found in Tables 3.4 and 3.5.

Aspirin is not routinely used as an analgesic in infants and children because of the risk of Reye's syndrome associated with its use in this population and is not a preferred analgesic in pediatrics. The most widely used mild analgesic for children is acetaminophen. The recommended weight-based dosing of acetaminophen in children is based on the dose response for antipyretic effects. Currently,

Table 3.4 Nonopioid Analgesics for the Relief of Pain in Neonates, Infants, and Children

Medicine	Dose (Oral Route)			Maximum Daily Dose
	Neonates (0 to 29 days)	Infants (30 days to 3 months)	Infants (3 to 12 months) or Children (1 to 12 years)[a,b]	
Paracetamol (also known as acetaminophen)	5–10 mg/kg every 6–8 h[a]	10 mg/kg every 4–6 h[a]	10–15 mg/kg every 4–6 h	Neonates, infants, and children: 4 doses/day
Ibuprofen			5–10 mg/kg every 6–8 h	Child: 40 mg/kg/day

[a] Children who are malnourished or in a poor nutritional state are more likely to be susceptible to toxicity at standard dose regimens because of a reduced natural detoxifying glutathione enzyme.

[b] Maximum of 1 g at a time.

From World Health Organization (WHO). Guidelines on the pharmacological treatment of persisting pain in children with medical illnesses. Geneva, Switzerland: WHO; 2012:41.

Table 3.5 Nonopioid Analgesics for the Relief of Pain in Neonates, Infants, and Children

Medicine	Dose (Oral Route)			Maximum Daily Dose
	Neonates (0 to 29 days)	Infants (30 days to 3 months)	Infants (3 to 12 months) or Children (1 to 12 years)[a,b]	
Paracetamol (also known as acetaminophen)	5–10 mg/kg every 6–8 h[a]	10 mg/kg every 4–6 h[a]	10–15 mg/ kg every 4–6 h	Neonates, infants, and children: 4 doses/day
Ibuprofen			5–10 mg/kg every 6–8 h	Child: 40 mg/kg/day

[a] Children who are malnourished or in a poor nutritional state are more likely to be susceptible to toxicity at standard dose regimens because of a reduced natural detoxifying glutathione enzyme.

[b] Maximum of 1 g at a time.

From World Health Organization (WHO). Guidelines on the pharmacological treatment of persisting pain in children with medical illnesses. Geneva, Switzerland: WHO; 2012:41.

there are no safety data on long-term acetaminophen use in children. NSAIDs have been shown to be safe and effective analgesics for children. Children using NSAIDs have been shown to have greater weight-normalized clearance and volumes of distribution than adults but with similar drug half-lives.

Use of Opioids in Children

There are now significant data supporting the use of specific opioids in children and adolescents.[1,31,32] It takes until age 2 to 6 months for the

Table 3.6 Starting Dosages for Opioid Analgesics in Opioid-Naïve Neonates

Medicine	Route of Administration	Starting Dose
Morphine	IV injection[a]	25–50 mcg/kg every 6 h
	SC injection	
	IV infusion	Initial IV dose[a] 25–50 mcg/kg, then 5–10 mcg/kg/h
		100 mcg/kg every 6 or 4 h
Fentanyl	IV injection[b]	1–2 mcg/kg every 2–4 h[c]
	IV infusion[b]	Initial IV dose 1–2 mcg/kg, then 0.5–1 mcg/ kg/h

[a] Administer IV morphine slowly over at least 5 minutes.

[b] The intravenous doses for neonates are based on acute pain management and sedation dosing information. Lower doses are required for nonventilated neonates.

[c] Administer IV fentanyl slowly over 3 to 5 minutes.

From World Health Organization (WHO). Guidelines on the pharmacological treatment of persisting pain in children with medical illnesses. Geneva, Switzerland: WHO; 2012:48.

Table 3.7 Starting Dosages for Opioid Analgesics in Opioid-Naïve Infants (1 Month to 1 Year)

Medicine	Route of Administration	Starting Dose
Morphine	Oral (immediate release)	80−200 mcg/kg every 4 h
	IV injection[a]	*1−6 mo:* 100 mcg/kg every 6 h
	SC injection	*6−12 mo:* 100 mcg/kg every 4 h (max: 2.5 mg/dose)
	IV infusion[a]	*1−6 mo:* initial IV dose 50 mcg/kg, then 10−30 mcg/kg/h *6−12 mo:* initial IV dose 100−200 mcg/kg, then 20−30 mcg/kg/h
	SC infusion	*1−3 mo:* 10 mcg/kg/h *3−12 mo:* 20 mcg/kg/h
Fentanyl[b]	IV injection	1−2 mcg/kg every 2−4 h[c]
	IV infusion	Initial IV dose 1−2 mcg/kg,[c] then 0.5−1 mcg/kg/h
Oxycodone	Oral (immediate release)	50−125 mcg/kg every 4 h

[a] Administer IV morphine slowly over at least 5 minutes.

[b] The intravenous doses for infants are based on acute pain management and sedation dosing information. Lower doses are required for nonventilated neonates.

[c] Administer IV fentanyl slowly over 3 to 5 minutes.

From World Health Organization (WHO). Guidelines on the pharmacological treatment of persisting pain in children with medical illnesses. Geneva, Switzerland: WHO; 2012:48.

weight-normalized clearance of many opioids to reach mature levels. Pharmacokinetic studies of morphine show an average serum half-life of 9 hours in preterm neonates, decreasing to 6.5 hours in full-term neonates and finally reaching 2 hours in the older infant. If not carefully monitored, neonates may be more likely to develop side effects from morphine due to decreased renal clearance of metabolites. The respiratory reflex response to hypoxemia, hypercapnia, and airway obstruction does not reach full maturity until 2 to 3 months after birth in both full-term and preterm infants. This can lead the nonintubated neonate receiving opioids to be at higher risk for respiratory depression. Neonates receiving opioids or other agents that can compromise cardiorespiratory function must be continuously monitored in a setting equipped to provide airway management. Those receiving prolonged opioid therapy may benefit from the use of continuous infusions to avoid the variation in plasma concentrations that occurs with bolus dosing. In neonates receiving synthetic opioids, the administration of infusions over several minutes or of small, frequent aliquots is recommended to avoid the adverse effects of glottic and chest wall rigidity that are associated with rapid bolus injection of medications such as fentanyl and sufentanil.

When using opioids with infants, children, and adolescents, the goal is to control pain as safely and quickly as possible. It is important to avoid repeated

Table 3.8 Starting Doses for Opioid Analgesics in Opioid-Naïve Children (1 to 12 Years)

Medicine	Route of Administration	Starting Dose
Morphine	Oral (immediate release)	1−2 y: 200−400 mcg/kg every 4 h 2−12 y: 200−500 mcg/kg every 4 h (max: 5 mg)
	Oral (prolonged release)	200−800 mcg/kg every 12 h
	IV injection[a]	1−2 y: 100 mcg/kg every 4 h
	SC injection	2−12 y: 100−200 mcg/kg every 4 h (max: 2.5 mg)
	IV infusion	Initial IV dose 100−200 mcg/kg,[a] then 20−30 mcg/kg/h
	SC infusion	20 mcg/kg/h
Fentanyl	IV injection	1−2 mcg/kg,[b] repeated every 30−60 min
	IV infusion	Initial IV dose 1−2 mcg/kg,[b] then 1 mcg/h
Hydromorphone[c]	Oral (immediate release)	30−80 mcg/kg every 3−4 h (max: 2 mg/dose)
	IV injection[d] or SC injection	15 mcg/kg every 3−6 h
Methadone[e]	Oral (immediate release)	100−200 mcg/kg every 4 h for the first 2−3 doses, then every 6−12 h (max: 5 mg/dose initially)[f]
	IV injection[g] and SC injection	
Oxymorphone	Oral (immediate release)	125−200 mcg/kg every 4 h (max: 5 mg/dose)
	Oral (prolonged release)	5 mg every 12 h

[a] Administer IV morphine slowly over at least 5 minutes.

[b] Administer IV fentanyl slowly over 3 to 5 minutes.

[c] Hydromorphone is a potent opioid, and significant differences exist between oral and intravenous dosing. Use extreme caution when converting from one route to another. In converting from parenteral hydromorphone to oral hydromorphone, doses may need to be titrated up to 5 times the IV dose.

[d] Administer IV hydromorphone slowly over 2 to 3 minutes.

[e] Because of the complex nature and wide interindividual variation in the pharmacokinetics of methadone, methadone should only be commenced by practitioners experienced in its use.

[f] Methadone should initially be titrated like other strong opioids. The dosage may need to be reduced by 50% 2 to 3 days after the effective dose has been found to prevent adverse effects because of methadone accumulation. From then on, dosage increases should be performed at intervals of 1 week or more, with a maximum dose increase of 50%.

[g] Administer IV methadone slowly over 3 to 5 minutes.

From World Health Organization (WHO). Guidelines on the pharmacological treatment of persisting pain in children with medical illnesses. Geneva, Switzerland: WHO; 2012:49.

administration of small, ineffective doses, which may prolong pain and worsen pain-related anxiety. For moderate to severe pain, it is appropriate to use opioids, such as morphine, fentanyl, hydromorphone, and methadone, in optimal doses titrated to an individual child's response.[1] Initial pediatric opioid dosing guidelines can be found in Tables 3.6, 3.7, and 3.8, . Meperidine, an opioid with a neurotoxic metabolite, should be avoided in pediatric patients.[1]

Patient-Controlled Analgesia by Proxy

Any discussion of opioid use in pediatrics would not be complete without a review of "patient-controlled analgesia (PCA) by proxy" and "authorized agent–controlled analgesia," or AACA. PCA is well established as a safe, effective method of pain control for children with moderate to severe pain in a variety of situations, including children in the last week of life. The risk for respiratory depression is lower because a sedated patient is less likely to press the demand button. PCA by proxy allows a person other than the patient to push the demand button. In 2004, the Joint Commission on Accreditation for Healthcare issued an alert regarding this practice, and in 2005, the Institute for Safe Medical Practices also issued a sentinel alert advising against this practice. The challenge is that some children who are unable to push the dose button by themselves would benefit from use of a PCA. Anghelescu and colleagues[33(p1625)] identified four groups of patients who would benefit from AACA. They include those unable to control a PCA pump because of: (1) age (usually <5 years) or cognitive ability; (2) neuromuscular impairment; (3) the need to undergo a painful procedure; and (4) end of life. These children are often opioid tolerant. The literature and the American Society for Pain Management Nursing advocate for AACA as a means of safe, effective pain control, when a designated proxy is carefully chosen and educated about appropriate use of PCA for the child.[5,33]

Use of Adjuvant Analgesics in Children

Adjuvant analgesics are a heterogeneous group of medications that include psychostimulants, corticosteroids, anticonvulsants, antidepressants, radionuclides, and neuroleptics. Much of the evidence supporting their use in specific targeted pain syndromes comes from the adult literature. Although gabapentin has been studied as an anticonvulsant in children, it has yet to be investigated as an adjuvant analgesic in children despite widespread use as such.[1] It is recommended that a child have baseline hematologic and biochemical laboratory studies and an electrocardiogram performed to rule out Wolff-Parkinson-White syndrome and other cardiac conduction defects before initiation of tricyclic antidepressants and at periodic intervals if the child receives long-term therapy or exceeds standard dose and weight guidelines.[34] Ketamine, a phencyclidine derivative, has been established as a useful medication to consider for procedural sedation and analgesia, when used by individuals who are trained in pediatric analgesia in pediatric settings[35,36] Future research on the use of adjuvant analgesics in the pediatric population is needed.

Use of Local Anesthetics and Other Anesthetic Techniques

In the past, local anesthetics were not widely used in children because of concerns regarding cardiac depression and seizures. Today, they are administered by a variety of routes and have an acceptable safety profile.

The use of regional nerve blocks in anesthetized children to provide improved postoperative analgesia has expanded during the past 20 years and been shown to be both effective and safe. This technique, which involves the injection of long-acting bupivacaine or ropivacaine into nerves that innervate a designated area, can also be used to provide local anesthesia for surgical procedures such as circumcision or reduction of fractures.[37]

Long-acting anesthetics (e.g., bupivacaine, ropivacaine) can be given intraspinally (epidurally or intrathecally) in children. Administration of epidural medications (opioids, local anesthetics, clonidine) can effectively control pain in children, including preterm neonates.[38] These medication are often given for postoperative pain control after specific procedures or in children with chronic pain who have not tolerated or responded well to systemic therapy.[37]

Nonpharmacologic Management

Nonpharmacologic pain management interventions include psychological, physiatric, neurostimulatory, invasive, and integrative techniques. Components are frequently combined as part of a pediatric pain management plan; they are dependent on the comprehensive pain assessment of an individual child and are based on the presumed etiology of pain.

In considering which nonpharmacologic interventions might be beneficial, the nurse needs to look at several factors, including the child's and family's past experience with nondrug interventions. What has worked well and what has not? Are there religious or cultural issues or concerns that would make certain interventions inappropriate? Is the proposed intervention consistent with the developmental level of the child? What is the present cognitive status of the child? Has the stress and fatigue from a prolonged illness made it difficult for the child or family members to concentrate, follow directions, or learn new information? Also, the nurse should consider teaching potentially useful techniques before the skills are needed.

Psychological interventions can include patient and family education, cognitive interventions, and behavioral techniques such as writing in a pain diary. Pain diaries may be especially useful in working with children who have recurrent or chronic pain, and their use has some value in pediatric pain research.[29] Children who enjoy writing may benefit from a private place to express themselves. Young children who have not mastered the written word may find drawing about their pain and pain experiences helpful.

The value of cognitive techniques such as distraction and relaxation is well established in children. A recent Cochrane review supports the emerging use of psychological therapies, primarily cognitive and behavioral therapies, to treat children with chronic or recurrent headache pain and nonheadache pain.[39] Another Cochrane review of the use of psychological nonpharmacologic techniques found sufficient evidence to recommend using techniques such as coaching, distraction, and hypnosis to help children cope with procedural pain. Across studies, distraction has been shown to reduce children's behavioral distress during procedural pain, although it has a variable effect on pain intensity. Various distractors have been used for children's pain management, including bubble-blowing, party blowers, puppetry, video games, and listening to music. The distractor is more likely to be effective if it is age appropriate and complementary to the interests and preferences of the individual child.

Procedural Pain Management

Procedural pain is a widespread experience for most children interacting with the healthcare system. Hospitalized children, who may or may not be dealing with a life-threatening illness, commonly undergo painful procedures. In a recent Canadian study of hospitalized children, 78% experienced a painful procedure within a 24-hour period before data collection.[40] Nurses who know how to successfully address procedural pain, using both pharmacologic and nonpharmacologic techniques, can help a very large number of children. Procedural pain is the one area in the pain literature that is much better developed for children than for adults, who may also experience this problem. The goals of successful procedural pain management include minimizing pain, maximizing patient cooperation, and minimizing risk to the patient[10]

Anticipation is the key word. Having procedures performed by technically competent individuals can reduce both risk for pain and risk for harm. The medical personnel involved must be knowledgeable in both pharmacologic and nonpharmacologic pain management appropriate to the child and the situation. Nonpharmacologic interventions can focus on the immediate environment and also on behavioral techniques.[10] Both children and parents need appropriate information regarding what will happen and how they can decrease stress.

Where Improvement Is Needed

All children are vulnerable to inadequate pain assessment and management. Those most vulnerable include the preverbal child, the cognitively or neurologically impaired child, immigrant children, and children without homes or consistent caregivers. Future work may need to look at the best ways to elicit symptoms such as pain, beyond the standard aspects of validity and reliability. Researchers need to clarify the effects of culture on the experience of pain in children.[9] System issues that interact with the barriers discussed earlier also need to be addressed (see Table 3.3).[1] For example, children cared for in pediatric tertiary care centers may find that healthcare professionals in their home environment lack up-to-date information about pain assessment and comprehensive pain control in children.

Pediatric groups are striving to achieve organizational changes in pediatric pain management. This can happen in many ways. In some settings, it involves creating a formal pediatric pain or palliative care service. In other settings, it may involve basic quality improvement programs. To start to improve the process of pain management, it is necessary to collect information about the present process, to develop an awareness of all the various factors that may either promote or deter achievement of the desired outcome. The literature reveals several efforts to collect baseline information about pain management and areas for improvement.[41] One area to consider is that of pain medication errors. Sources of errors in pediatric medication administration include dilution errors, milligram-microgram errors, decimal point errors, and confusion between a total daily dose and a fractional dose.[42,43] Through application of the quality improvement process, nurses can play an important role in improving pain control for both the individual children they care for and other children with whom they may not be directly involved.

Summary

Despite the significant increase in knowledge about assessment and management of pain in infants and children, too many suffering children do not receive proper treatment. In today's age of "powerful, invasive medicine, we can save more lives, but any wrong choice turns medicine into torture, inflicting avoidable sufferings on patients."[44(p2)] Pediatric palliative care exists to mitigate suffering in children with life-threatening illnesses.[30] To prevent suffering for children and their families, nurses and other healthcare professionals must apply the most up-to-date techniques of pain assessment and management to all children they care for, especially from the time a child receives a diagnosis of a potentially life-threatening illness through his or her survival or death. By application of an integrated treatment plan that is based on the developmental level of the individual child, involves his or her family, and uses both pharmacologic and nonpharmacologic interventions, optimal pain control is possible.

References

1. World Health Organization (WHO). Guidelines on the pharmacological treatment of persisting pain in children with medical illnesses. Geneva, Switzerland: WHO; 2012.

2. Pain terms: a list with definitions and notes on usage. Recommended by the International Association for the Study of Pain Subcommittee on Taxonomy. *Pain.* 1979;6:249-252.

3. McCaffery M, Pasero C. *Pain: Clinical Manual.* 2nd ed. St. Louis: Mosby; 1999.

4. Gauvain-Piquard A, Rodary C, Rezvani A, Serbouti S. The development of the DEGR®: a scale to assess pain in young children with cancer. *Eur J Pain.* 1999;2:165-176.

5. Knegt NC, Pieper MJC, Lobbezoo F, et al. Behavioral pain indicators in people with intellectual disabilities: a systematic review. *J Pain.* 2013;14(9):885-896.

6. Silva FC, Thuler LC. Cross-cultural adaption and translation of two pain assessment tools in children and adolescents. *J Pediatr.* 2008;84(4):344-349.

7. World Health Organization (WHO). *Cancer Pain Relief and Palliative Care in Children.* Geneva, Switzerland: WHO; 1998.

8. Collins JJ. Management of symptoms associated with cancer: pain management. In: Carroll WL, Finlay JL, eds. *Cancer in Children and Adolescents.* Sudbury, MA: Jones and Bartlett; 2009.

9. Ruland CM, Hamilton GA, Schjodt-Osmo B. The complexity of symptoms and problems experienced in children with cancer: a review of the literature. *J Pain Symptom Manage.* 2009;37(3):403-418.

10. Cramton REM, Gruchala NE. Managing procedural pain in pediatric patients. *Curr Opin Pediatr.* 2012;24(4):530-538.

11. Padhye B, Dalla-Pozza L, Little DG, Munns CF. Use of zoledronic acid for chemotherapy related osteonecrosis in children and adolescents: a retrospective analysis. *Pediatr Blood Cancer.* 2013;60:1539-1545.

12. American Pain Society (APS). *Guidelines for the Management of Acute and Chronic Pain in Sickle Cell Disease.* Glenview, IL: APS, 1999.

13. Russo R, Miller M, Haan E, et al. Pain characteristics and their association with quality of life and self-concept in children with hemiplegic cerebral palsy identified from a population register. *Clin J Pain.* 2008;24(4):335-342.

14. Hartley C, Slater R. Neurophysiological measures of nociceptive brain activity in the newborn infant: the next steps. *Acta Paediatr.* 2014;103(3):238-242.

15. American Academy of Pediatrics, Canadian Pediatric Society. Prevention and management of pain and stress in the neonate. *Pediatrics.* 2000;105:454-461.

16. Berde CB, Setna NF. Analgesics for the treatment of pain in children. *N Engl J Med.* 2003;347:1094-1103.

17. Lawrence J, Alcock D, McGrath P, et al. The development of a tool to assess neonatal pain expression. *Neonatal Netw.* 1993;12:59-66.

18. Krechel SW, Bildner J. CRIES: a new neonatal postoperative pain measurement tool. Initial testing of validity and reliability. *Paediatr Anaesth.* 1995;5:53-61.

19. Stevens BJ, Johnson C, Petryshen P, Taddio A. Premature infant pain profile: development and initial validation. *Clin J Pain.* 1996;12:13-22.

20. Grunau RVE, Craig KD. Facial activity as a measure of neonatal pain expression. In: Tyler EC, Krane EJ, eds. *Advances in Pain Research Therapy: Pediatric Pain.* Vol. 15. New York: Raven; 1990;147-155.

21. Levetown M, ed. *Compendium of Pediatric Palliative Care.* Alexandria, VA: National Hospice and Palliative Care Organization; 2000.

22. McGrath PJ, Johnson G, Goodman JT, et al. CHEOPS: a behavioral scale for rating postoperative pain in children. In: Fields HL, Dubner R, Cervero F, eds. *Advances in Pain Research and Therapy.* Vol. 9. New York: Raven; 1985;395-402.

23. Power N, Liossi C, Franck L. Helping parents to help their child with procedural and everyday pain: practical, evidence-based advice. J Spec Pediatr Nurs. 2007;12(3):203-209.

24. Davies B, Contro N, Larson J, Widger K. Culturally-sensitive information-sharing in pediatric palliative care. *Pediatrics.* 2010;125(4):e559-e865.

25. Jacob E, Mack AK, Savedra M, et al. Adolescent pediatric pain tool for multidimensional measurement of pain in children and adolescents. *Pain Manag Nurs.* 2014;15(3):694-706.

26. Levine D, Lam CG, Cunningham MJ, et al. Best practices for pediatric palliative care: a primer for clinical providers. *J Support Oncol.* 2013;11(3):114-125.

27. McGrath PA, Brown SC. Pain control. In: Doyle D, Hanks G, Cherny N, et al, eds. *Oxford Textbook of Palliative Medicine.* 3rd ed. New York: Oxford University Press; 2004.

28. Field MJ, Behrman R, eds. When Children Die: Improving Palliative and End-of-Life Care for Children and Their Families. Report of the Institute of Medicine Task Force. Washington, DC: National Academy Press; 2003

29. Jacob E. Pain assessment and management in children. In: Hockenberry MJ, Wilson D, eds. *Wong's Nursing Care of Infants and Children.* 9th ed. St Louis: Elsevier Mosby; 2011:179-226.

30. Baker C, Wong D. Q.U.E.S.T.: A process of pain assessment in children. *Orthop Nurs.* 1987;6:11-21.

31. Krekels EH, Tibboel D, Kanhof M, Knibbe CA. Prediction of morphine clearance in the paediatric population: how accurate are the available pharmacokinetic models? *Clin Pharmacokinet.* 2012;51(11):695-709.

32. Davies D, DeVlaming D, Haines C. Methadone analgesia for children with advanced cancer. *Pediatr Blood Cancer.* 2008;51(3):393-397.

33. Anghelescu D, Burgoyne L, Oakes L, Wallace D. The safety of patient-controlled analgesia by proxy in pediatric oncology patients. *Anesth Analg*. 2005;101:1623-1627.

34. Collins JJ, Berde CB, Frost JA. Pain assessment and management. In: Wolfe J, Hinds PS, Sourkes BM, eds. *Textbook of Interdisciplinary Pediatric Palliative Care*. Philadelphia: Elsevier Saunders: 2011:284-299.

35. Morton N. Ketamine for procedural sedation and analgesia in pediatric emergency medicine: A UK perspective. *Paediatr Anaesth*. 2008;18:25-29.

36. Dallimore D, Herd D, Short T, Anderson B. Dosing ketamine for pediatric procedural sedation in the emergency room department. *Pediatr Emerg Care*. 2008;24(8):529-533.

37. Suresh S, Birmingham PK, Kozlowski RJ. Pediatric pain management. *Anesthesiol Clin*. 2012;30:101-117.

38. Bosenberg A, Flick RP. Regional anesthesia in neonates and infants. *Clin Perinatol*. 2013;40(3):525-538.

39. Eccleston C, Palerma TM, Williams ACDC, et al. Psychological therapies for the management of chronic and recurrent pain in children and adolescents (Review). *Cochrane Database Syst Rev*. 2013;8:1-81.

40. Stevens BJ, Abbott LK, Yamada J, et al. Epidemiology and management of painful procedures in children in Canadian hospitals. *Can Med Assoc J*. 2011;183:E403-E410.

41. Bigham MT, Schwartz HP; Ohio Neonatal/Pediatric Transport Quality Collaborative. *Pediatr Crit Med*. 2013;14(5):515-524.

42. Broussard L. Small size, big risk: preventing neonatal and pediatric medication errors. *Nurs Womens Health*. 2010;14(5):405-408

43. Tzimenatos L, Bond GR; Pediatric Therapeutic Error Study Group. Severe injury or death in young children from therapeutic errors: a summary of 238 cases from the American Association of Poison Control Centers. *Clin Toxicol*. 2009;47(4):348-354.

44. Facco E, Giron G. The nature of pain and the approach to the suffering child. Suffering Child. 2003;2(February):1-3. Available at http://www.the suffering child.net Accessed February 28, 2005.

Chapter 4

Palliative Care in the Neonatal Intensive Care Unit

Cheryl Thaxton, Brigit Carter, and Chi Dang Hornik

For several years, a substantial effort has been made to adequately address the needs of neonatal palliative care patients and families. Parents face months of anguish as they prepare for the birth of a child with a suspected lethal congenital anomaly. The sudden delivery of a prematurely born infant can also pose existential reflections within the family unit. The answer to what was a predictable and planned future suddenly can become uncertain and overwhelming. Grandparents and extended family members often stand by in search of the "right things to say" to support the situation. Siblings are in the midst of the deep sense of confusion, during what was once a time of anticipation; as the time draws near for the birth of the baby, each family member will transition through thoughts that pose more questions than answers. Families may find it hard to acknowledge that the infant has an incurable condition, thus creating a barrier to accessing palliative care measures.[1]

American society does not have a word for a parent who has lost a child. For example, the term *widow* is used for the surviving female spouse, but what do we call the surviving parent? Other cultures may have words or strategies to support parents who have lost an infant, but American culture labels the person a bereaved parent and refers to another child in the parents' future or another living child.

This chapter presents the core values of neonatal palliative care, within the context of providing culturally appropriate, compassionate, individualized, family-centered developmental care (IFCDC) and patient-focused care for infants in the neonatal intensive care unit (NICU) environment. To illustrate use of palliative care with the neonatal population, the following case study was supplied by a parent.

Case Study: In Utero With Congenital Diaphragmatic Hernia

Dylan was diagnosed in utero with congenital diaphragmatic hernia (CDH) at 16 weeks by ultrasound (this section is written entirely by his family).

> Knowing about his CDH during pregnancy gave us time to adjust to the news and learn all this medical stuff, so when Dylan was born we could

totally focus on him and be very present/in the moment. One objective during our pregnancy was to bond with Dylan. We wanted him to know and feel that we loved him, we wanted him and we would do everything we could to help him live. So we constantly talked to him. We thought this bonding was what we could do, our part to help when he was born. We grew to love the monthly ultrasounds. It was another way to further bond with Dylan. We were amazed at the amount of detail we could see—hair, eyelashes, nose, mouth, chin. We realize we saw him more active in the ultrasounds (e.g., swallow, suck thumb, hand pulled on ear and foot) than after he was born.

I *knew* Dylan could die, but I had to totally believe he would live. Sometimes I would think about him dying. I cried and tried to get it out of my system. I did not want to *feel* he could die because if I could feel that, then Dylan could. And I did not want Dylan to feel he could die. Not having control or knowing the outcome was frustrating. As my due date drew nearer, I was scared because soon we'd know the outcome. But as frustrating as the unknown was, Dylan was safe during that time while he was in me—he was "healthy," alive, and kicking. It was only going to be when he was born that he'd be critically sick. I wanted to keep him in me to keep him safe.

We talked to the specialists who might be involved in Dylan's care about possible outcomes. We always got to one path where there was no progress and the machines would be what were keeping him alive. I hoped it would not get to that point. I did not think I could make the decision to let Dylan die. We got the same story from everybody (OBs/surgeon/NICU/PICU) regarding a CDH. It was good to get the same message, nothing was conflicting. But it was very depressing, we always got hit with reality. No rosy picture was painted.

Dylan was born and placed on extracorporeal membrane oxygenation (ECMO). After we went to our room, the PICU physician visited a few times with updates; unfortunately, none of it was good news. We went through all the ventilation options, and ECMO was the next and only remaining step. Did we want to proceed? Yes, we expected to give Dylan every opportunity to live. We realized later that we may not have been good at communicating this upfront.

It was great to have access to the room across from the NICU to sleep. Even though we only live 10 minutes from the hospital, it was 10 minutes too far. It felt like 1,000 miles away. It was good to stay over, particularly after Dylan's surgery. When we went home at night, we were always afraid we would get a call in the middle of the night from the PICU saying Dylan had died. I couldn't bear the thought of him dying alone, all by himself.

It took me a few days to realize I had not heard a sound out of Dylan, not a peep, not a cry. And I wouldn't until the ventilator tube was removed. Up until then, my usual reaction when I heard a baby screaming was to cringe and hope the parents could quickly quiet their child. Now, Dylan's cries would be music to my ears.

Dylan turned 2 weeks old. Those 2 weeks allowed us to get to know Dylan and be his parents. We enjoyed every little thing, and most of them were simple, subtle things. Dylan's face was swollen, and he struggled for days to open his eyes. He finally opened his right one. It felt so good that he got to see us, and his eye was so expressive. Sometimes it was very curious, looking all around. Another time it pierced my heart when he was unhappy with something they were doing to him. His look was like, "Mom, how can you let them do this to me?" We could tell how strong he was when he gripped our fingers in his hands. I loved that Dylan was such a fighter. I was so proud of him. We were constantly talking to and touching Dylan. When we were told Dylan had too much stimulation, we had to just sit and watch him. That was difficult. We told Dylan that we were there with him, even if he couldn't hear or feel us. That gave me time to just adore him and look at all of his features.

It felt great that both NICU and PICU staff told us Dylan recognized our voices. They said it did not happen with our other family members present, only with his father and me. We were so happy that Dylan knew us, and we seemed to have a positive effect on him. Comments were made that it must be hard for us because each day we were bonding and getting more attached to Dylan. We never thought of it that way. What we were doing, just being with him and loving him, was easy. You just can't turn off this love that is gushing out of you. What else would we do? How could any parent not be with their baby every minute they could? Again, the idea was to bond with Dylan. If he could feel all of our love for him, maybe that could carry him through. We never considered pulling away from Dylan because we thought he might die. I would never be able to forgive myself if I wasn't with him or stopped loving him. Was our attachment to Dylan noticeable because it contrasted the detachment of medicine? I kissed Dylan on his head and told him I loved him every time I left his room; I could never kiss him and tell him I loved him too much. In case something happened when I was away, I would know those were my last words to him.

We would see the medical students gather for rounds. One would come in Dylan's room and pull numbers from his chart. They never talked to us and never once stopped to even look at Dylan. We wondered how did they learn about the human side of medicine. How did they learn to interact with patients and families? How did they learn compassionate care? We continued to learn about the human body and medicine. Such a delicate balance is required. Dylan needed to do seemingly opposite things to get better. *When I took a breath I would think, this was "all" we were trying to get him to do.*

Dylan had his surgery to repair his CDH while on ECMO. Dylan was being weaned off ECMO. We heard optimism from the docs. I think for the first time even the docs thought Dylan might pull through, but over the next few weeks, the physicians noted not much improvement, and Dylan was in multi-organ system failure. It was made very clear that there was no more optimism, and in fact just the opposite was now true, Dylan would continue to deteriorate. We decided to give ourselves some time for that to sink in before we made any decisions.

That afternoon we were told that it was affecting his heart (it had been strong up until then). Now we had to let him go. The machines could have kept him alive for a while longer, but that was not best for Dylan. As much as we wanted more time with him, letting him die in peace and with dignity was more important. I am surprised at how "easy" it was; my husband and I barely had a conversation about it, we knew what we had to do. All I could think was—I finally was going to get to hold Dylan.

That last night we stayed up all night with Dylan. In the middle of the night I asked the respiratory therapist to suction him. She asked if I wanted to and I said yes. It felt really good to do that. Then she asked if we wanted to give him a sponge bath and we said yes. So my husband and I cleaned him up and then put lotion all over him. Doing all of these things for Dylan made me so happy but I had no idea why. What was the big deal? I was just giving him a bath. Later I figured it out. I got to be a Mom and take care of Dylan. I got to do some of the things I had planned to do with him at home.

When Dylan was getting prepped for us to hold, the nurse asked whether we had Dylan's footprints and handprints. I said I didn't think so, I had not seen them if they were done. So she did that, and we cut some locks of his hair. I had not thought of these things at all. I am so glad she did.

There are no words to describe the feelings when we finally got to hold Dylan. My husband told me later it was the first time he saw me truly relax since we had gotten Dylan's diagnosis. It was wonderful for our little family to be so close together. It was the first time the three of us were alone. It was very comforting that Dylan could die in our arms.

Case Summary

"As much as we wanted more time with him, letting him die in peace and with dignity was more important." "It was very comforting that Dylan could die in our arms." These words, as stated by Dylan's parents, echo the true essence of neonatal palliative care. Parents are faced with challenging decisions and even some uncertainties in shifting focus from curative therapies to palliative care measures.[2] Providing a seamless transition into palliative care requires support and an interdisciplinary effort by the entire healthcare team. The team focus should be to provide optimal conditions for the infant's life and death, including interventions to prevent and relieve suffering.[2] Implementing a palliative care protocol involves tremendous flexibility that supports a variety of choices, moving in and out of active life-sustaining measures, until the end of the infant's life. The nurse plays a vital role in ensuring that communication with the family is not fragmented, that parents are reassured that the best effort will be made to support their wishes throughout the uncertainty of the journey. Dignity should be maintained at all costs. Patient- and family-centered care measures seek to ensure that a dying infant's final hours are spent in a peaceful environment, in the presence of the family.

Standard of Care for Neonatal Patients

The care of the neonatal palliative care patient is not setting-specific. Care can be provided within the NICU, in a newborn special care unit, or through a perinatal home hospice program. The nurse is instrumental in providing goal-directed support that integrates curative therapies with palliative measures. Extremely premature infants with multiple comorbidities are potential candidates for neonatal palliative care. Because of the high morbidity and mortality rates for extremely premature infants, many expectant parents are confronted during the prenatal period with the possibility that their infant may be too small for resuscitation to take place in the delivery room.[3] To deliver care that is interdisciplinary as well as patient and family-centered, nurses work alongside neonatologists, nurse practitioners, social workers, geneticists, respiratory therapists, pharmacists, and many subspecialists.

Nurses can take part in neonatal palliative care discussions when there is a consultative palliative care team or specialist involved. Nurses often lead communication with the family because they spend the most time with the infant. Wigert, Dellenmark, and Bry reported a quantitative and a qualitative analysis of strengths and weaknesses perceived by parents in their communication with doctors and nurses at the NICU.[4] The study noted that communication with nurses was described as a source of emotional support more often than communication with doctors. Nurses, because of the nature of their job, are more often at the bedside and thus are more available for emotional contact with families.[4] Parents and caregivers often voice concerns to the bedside nurse as they process difficult information about the infant's medical status. The neonatal nurse should be prepared to provide palliative care support within the context of the infant's trajectory while addressing issues of uncertainty with the support of the interdisciplinary care team (Table 4.1).

The Family as the Unit of Care

The case study demonstrates the importance of providing comfort care measures to support the end of life care experiences of the patient and family (Box 4.1). The nurse has to be present at the most difficult time for the family, fully attentive to the child and family, able to separate personal values regarding birth, life, and death from those of the family. Nurses must adapt and individualize the care, so that there is as much support for the positive development, as possible, for the infant and family. An IFCDC approach provides the context in which to render palliative and end of life care. The nurse is reminded that within the family unit, parents are first; they want to support their infant's development and preserve their role as parents. It is only after the parental role is solidified that parents can become the caregivers to a child that may or will die. For culturally competent care, the nurse must be properly prepared to be sensitive to the family's cultural, ethnic, and religious values.

Cultural Influences on Care

Cultural values and beliefs, both religious and ethnic, influence the family's view of pain, suffering, and end of life (Table 4.2). The neonatal nurse must incorporate these values and beliefs into the plan of care if it is to be effective

Table 4.1 Ethical Principles and Application to Perinatal Palliative Care

Ethical Principle	Definition	Application to Perinatal Palliative Care
Autonomy	The principle of self-determination in which patients participate in decisions about their lives	Provide and clarify the parents' understanding of case-specific information. Ensure informed consent.
Beneficence and nonmaleficence	The principle placing the patient's best interest first and the principle duty to first "do no harm" dictates obligation to protect patient safety and not cause injury	Identify values that each family brings to the situation; respect wishes, clarify treatment options (or lack thereof), and use bioethical principles to guide conversations.
Justice	The principle that means to give each person or group what is "due"	Ensure equitable access to care and resources, including access to staff members; palliative care protocols and support should be implemented by clinicians and supported by administrators.
Dignity	The principle that every human has intrinsic worth	The mother, fetus, and family have the right to be treated with respect and honor.
Truthfulness and honesty	The principle of veracity in which the clinician provides information regarding diagnosis and care alternatives	Recognize that some clinical scenarios involve irresolvable tragedies. Conduct an assessment of patient knowledge and offer truthful information in a compassionate, gentle, and sensitive manner.

Adapted from Wool C. Clinician confidence and comfort in providing perinatal palliative care. J Obstet Gynecol Neonat Nurs. 2013;42(1):48-58.[5]

and of benefit to the patient and family. Hockenberry and Wilson[7] and the Texas Children's Cancer Center–Texas Children's Hospital[8] address cultural influence on care by outlining key aspects of health beliefs and practices that must be considered when providing any type of care.

For example, when working with a Native American family, the nurse must consider how to combine healing ceremonies from their tribal rituals with Western medicine to alleviate suffering. In this instance, ethnic and religious beliefs are intertwined. But in other instances, religious and ethnic values must be differentiated and incorporated into care. Not every family that identifies with an organized religion strictly adheres to all principles of that faith. One example of religious belief affecting neonatal palliative care is that of an American Caucasian family strongly tied to the Catholic Church. As their infant girl took a turn for the worst, the family was called. They immediately asked that she be baptized. The priest on call was unavailable, and the family's

> **Box 4.1 Core Concepts of Patient- and Family-Centered Care**
>
> - **Dignity and respect.** Healthcare practitioners listen to and honor patient and family perspectives and choices. Patient and family knowledge, values, beliefs, and cultural backgrounds are incorporated into the planning and delivery of care.
> - **Information sharing.** Healthcare practitioners communicate and share complete and unbiased information with patients and families in ways that are affirming and useful. Patients and families receive timely, complete, and accurate information to effectively participate in care and decision-making.
> - **Participation.** Patients and families are encouraged and supported in participating in care and decision-making at the level they choose.
> - **Collaboration.** Patients, families, healthcare practitioners, and leaders collaborate in policy and program development, implementation, and evaluation; in healthcare facility design; in professional education; and in the delivery of care.
>
> Adapted from the Institute for Patient- and Family-Centered Care, 2013; http://www.ipfcc. org/. Reprinted with permission.[6]

priest was 2 hours away. Rather than take the chance that no priest would come before the infant's death, the nurse, a non-Catholic, baptized the baby. When the family arrived, they were reassured that Angela had been baptized. The infant died peacefully in her parents' arms, long before either priest arrived. The family expressed comfort in knowing she was held within the religious arms of the Church's beliefs.

Catlin[9] studied 684 infants with life-threatening or chronic illnesses. She found that many infants stay 6 months or longer in the hospital and that 20% of NICU infants are transferred to a pediatric intensive care unit (PICU) to die, even when care will most likely be futile. Thus, despite having a palliative care protocol[10] supported at a national level, dissemination to individual institutions or units has not occurred. Nurses suffered moral distress as they were required to render futile and sometimes painful care.[9] As Anand suggests, healthcare professionals must also understand current pharmacologic treatment of pain and use the most effective methods tailored to the individual infant to alleviate distress.[11]

Recognizing Differences in Palliative Care

Most neonatal health professionals recognize the unique needs of this population, including their rights and their care needs. An infant has no history—as one family said, the infant does not know what the future possibilities are; there is no frame of reference. For the family, there are no memories of a past except prenatally, so palliative care is building a lifetime of memories. Box 4.2 summarizes other differences. The nurse should become familiar with the patient's disease-specific needs and address the family's needs

Table 4.2 Religious Influences

Religious Sect	Birth	Death	Organ Donation/Transplantation	Beliefs Regarding Medical Care
Baptist	Infant baptism is not practiced. However, many churches present the baby and the parents to the congregation when they attend services for the first time after the birth.	It is not mandatory that clergy be present at death, but families often desire visits from clergy. Scripture reading and prayer are important.	There is no formal statement regarding this issue. It is considered a matter of personal conscience. It is commonly regarded as positive (an act of love).	Some may regard their illness as punishment resulting from past sins. Those who believe in predestination may not seek aggressive treatment. Fundamentalist and conservative groups see the Bible as the infallible word of God to be taken literally.
Buddhist	Do not practice infant baptism.	Buddhist priest is often involved before and after death. Rituals are observed during and after death. If the family does not have a priest, they may request that one be contacted.	There is no formal statement regarding organ donation/transplantation. This is seen as a matter of individual conscience.	Believe that illness can be used as a tool to aid in the development of the soul. May see illness as a result of karmic causes. May avoid treatments or procedures on holy days. Cleanliness is important.
Church of Jesus Christ of Latter-Day Saints (Mormon)	Infant baptism is not performed. Children are given a name and a priesthood blessing sometime after the birth, from 1–2 weeks to several months. In the event of a critically ill newborn, this might be done in the hospital at the discretion of the parents. Baptism is performed after the child is 8 years old. Members of Church of Jesus Christ of Latter-Day Saints feel that a child is not accountable for sins before 8 years of age.	There are no religious rituals performed related to death.	There is no official statement regarding this issue. Organ donation/transplantation is left up to the individual or parents.	Administration to the sick involves anointing with consecrated oil and performing a blessing by members of the priesthood. Although the individual or a member of the family usually requests this if the individual is unconscious and there is no one to represent him or her, it would be appropriate for anyone to contact the Church so that the ordinance may be performed. Refusal of medical treatments would be left up to the individual. There are no restrictions relative to "holy" days.

Episcopal	Infant baptism is practiced. In emergency situations, request for infant baptism should be given high priority and could be performed by any baptized person, clergy, or layperson. Often, in situations of stillbirths or aborted fetuses, special prayers of commendation may be offered.	Pastoral care of the sick may include prayers, laying on of hands, anointing, and/ or Holy Communion. At the time of death, various litanies and special prayers may be offered.	Both are permitted.	Respect for the dignity of the whole person is important. These needs include physical, emotional, and spiritual.
Society of Friends (Quakers)	Do not practice infant baptism.	Each person has a divine nature, but an encounter and relationship with Jesus Christ is essential.	No formal statement, but generally both are permitted.	No special rites or restrictions. Leaders and elders from the Church may visit and offer support and encouragement. Quakers believe in plain speech.
Islam (Muslim/ Moslem)	At birth, the first words said to the infant in his/her right ear are "Allah-o-Akbar" (Allah is great), and the remainder of the Call for Prayer is recited. An Aqeeqa (party) to celebrate the birth of the child is arranged by the parents. Circumcision of the male child is practiced.	In Islam, life is meant to be a test for the preparation for everlasting life in the hereafter. Therefore, according to Islam, death is simply a transition. Islam teaches that God has prescribed the time of death for everyone and only He knows when, where, or how a person is going to die. Islam encourages making the best use of all of God's gifts, including the precious gift of life in this world. At the time of death, there are specific rituals (e.g., bathing, wrapping the body in cloth) that must be done. Before moving and handling the body, it is preferable to contact someone from the person's mosque or Islamic Society to perform these rituals.	Permitted. However, there are some stipulations depending on the type of transplant/donation and its effect on the donor and recipient. It is advisable to contact the individual's mosque or the local Islamic Society for further consultation.	Humans are encouraged in the Qur'an (Koran) to seek treatment. It is taught that only Allah cures. However, Muslims are taught not to refuse treatment in the belief that Allah will take care of them because even though He cures, He also chooses at times to work through the efforts of humans.

(continued)

Table 4.2 (Continued)

Religious Sect	Birth	Death	Organ Donation/Transplantation	Beliefs Regarding Medical Care
International Society for Krishna Consciousness (a Hindu movement in North America based on devotion to Lord Krishna)	Infant baptism is not performed.	The body should not be touched. The family may desire that a local temple be contacted so that representatives may visit and chant over the patient. It is believed that in chanting the names of God, one may gain insight and God consciousness.	There is no formal statement prohibiting this act. It is an individual decision.	Illness or injury is believed to represent sins committed in this or a previous life. They accept modern medical treatment. The body is seen as a temporary vehicle used to transport them through this life. The body belongs to God, and members are charged to care for it in the best way possible.
Jehovah's Witnesses	Infant baptism is not practiced.	There are no official rites that are performed before or after death; however, the faith community is often involved and supportive of the patient and family.	There is no official statement related to this issue. Organ donation is not encouraged, but it is believed to be an individual decision. According to the legal corporation for the denomination, Watchtower, all donated organs and tissue must be drained of blood before transplantation.	Adherents are absolutely opposed to transfusions of whole blood, packed red blood cells, platelets, and fresh or frozen plasma. This includes banking of ones' own blood. Many accept use of albumin, globulin, factor replacement (hemophilia), vaccines, hemodilution, and cell salvage. There is no opposition to nonblood plasma expanders.
Judaism (Orthodox and Conservative)	Circumcision of male infants is performed on the 8th day if the infant is healthy. The mohel (ritual circumciser familiar with Jewish law and aseptic technique) performs the ritual.	It is important that the healthcare professional facilitate the family's need to comfort and be with the patient at the time of death.	Permitted and is considered a mitzvah (good deed).	Only emergency surgical procedures should be performed on the Sabbath, which extends from sundown Friday to sundown Saturday. Elective surgery should be scheduled for days other than the Sabbath. Pregnant women and the seriously ill are exempt from fasting. Serious illness may be grounds for violating dietary laws but only if it is medically necessary.

Lutheran	Infant baptism is practiced. If the infant's prognosis is poor, the family may request immediate baptism.	Family may desire visitation from clergy. Prayers for the dying, commendation of the dying, and prayers for the bereaved may be offered.	There is no formal statement regarding this issue. It is considered a matter of personal conscience.	Illness is not seen as an act of God; rather, it is seen as a condition of humankind's fallen state. Prayers for the sick may be desired.
Methodist	Infant baptism is practiced but is usually done within the community of the Church after counseling and guidance from clergy. However, in emergency situations, a request for baptism would not be seen as inappropriate.	In the case of perinatal death, there are prayers within the United Methodist Book of worship that could be said by anyone. Prayer, scripture, and singing are often seen as appropriate and desirable.	Organ donation/transplantation is supported and encouraged. It is considered a part of good stewardship.	In the Methodist tradition, it is believed that every person has the right to death with dignity and has the right to be involved in all medical decisions. Refusal of aggressive treatment is seen as an appropriate option.
Pentecostal Assembly of God, Church of God, Four Square, and many other faith groups are included under this general heading. Pentecostal is not a denomination, but a theologic distinctive (pneumatology).	No rituals such as baptism are necessary. Many Pentecostals have a ceremony of "dedication," but it is done in the context of the community of faith/believers (the Church). Children belong to heaven and only become sinners after the age of accountability, which is not clearly defined.	The only way to transcend this life; it is the door to heaven (or hell). Questions about "salvation of the soul" are very common and important. Resurrection is the hope of those who "were saved." Prayer is appropriate; so are singing and scripture reading.	Many Pentecostal denominations have no statement concerning this subject, but it is generally seen as positive and well received. Education concerning wholeness of the person and nonliteral aspects like "heart" and "mind" have to be explained. For example, a Pentecostal may have a problem with donating a heart to a "nonbeliever."	Pentecostals are sometimes labeled as "in denial" because of their theology of healing. Their faith in God for literal healing is generally expressed as intentional unbelief in the prognostic statements. Many Pentecostals do not see sickness as the will of God; thus one must "stand firm" in faith and accept the unseen reality, which many times may mean healing. As difficult as this position may seem, it must be noted that, when death occurs, Pentecostals may leap from miracle expectations to joyful hope and theology of heaven and resurrection without facing issues of anger or frustration due to unfulfilled expectations. Prayer, scriptures, singing, and anointing of the sick (not a sacrament) are appropriate/expected pastoral interventions.

(continued)

Table 4.2 (Continued)

Religious Sect	Birth	Death	Organ Donation/ Transplantation	Beliefs Regarding Medical Care
Presbyterian	Baptism is a sacrament of the Church but is not considered necessary for salvation. However, it is seen as an event to take place, when possible, in the context of a worshipping community.	Family may desire visitation from clergy. Prayers for the dying, commendation of the dying, and prayers for the bereaved may be offered.	There is no formal statement regarding this issue.	Communion is a sacrament of the Church. It is generally celebrated with a patient in the presence of an ordained minister and elder. Presbyterians are free to make their own choices regarding the use of mechanical life-support measures.
Roman Catholic	Infant baptism is practiced. In medical facilities, baptism is usually performed by a priest or deacon, as ordinary members of the sacrament. However, under extraordinary circumstances, baptism may be administered by a layperson, provided that the intention is to do as the Church does, using the formula, "I baptise you in the name of the Father, the Son, and the Holy Spirit."	Sacrament of the sick is the sacrament of healing and forgiveness. It is to be administered by a priest as early in the illness as possible. It is not a last rite to be administered at the point of death. The Roman Catholic Church makes provisions for prayers of commendation of the dying, which may be said by any priest, deacon, sacramental minister, or layperson.	Catholics may donate or receive organ transplants.	The Sacrament of Holy Communion sustains Catholics in sickness as in health. When the patient's condition deteriorates, the sacrament is given as viaticum ("food for the journey"). Like Holy Communion, viaticum may be administered by a priest, deacon, or sacramental minister. The Church makes provisions for prayers for commendation of the dying that may be said by any of those listed above or by a layperson.

Adapted from Texas Children's Cancer Center–Texas Children's Hospital. End-of-Life Care for Children. Houston: Texas Cancer Council; 2000[a]; and Wigert H, Dellenmark MB, Bry K. Strengths and weaknesses of parent–staff communication in the NICU: a survey assessment. BMC Pediatr. 2013;13:71.

Box 4.2 Differences Between Hospice Care for Newborns/ Infants and Adults

Patient Issues

- Patient is not legally competent.
- Patient is in developmental process that affects understanding of life and death, sickness and health, God, and so forth.
- Patient has not achieved a "full and complete life."
- Patient lacks verbal skills to describe needs, feelings, and so forth.
- Patient is often in a highly technical medical environment.

Family Issues

- Family needs to protect the child from information about his or her health.
- Family needs to do everything possible to save the child.
- Family may have difficulty dealing with siblings.
- Family feels stress on finances.
- Family fears that care at home is not as good as care at the hospital.
- Grandparents feel helpless in dealing with their children and grandchildren.
- Family needs relief from burden of care.

Caregiver Issues

- Caregivers need to protect children, parents, and siblings.
- Caregivers feel a sense of failure in not saving the child.
- Caregivers feel a sense of "ownership" of children, even at the expense of parents.
- Caregivers have out-of-date ideas about pain in children, especially infants.
- Caregivers lack knowledge about children's disease processes.
- Caregivers are influenced by "unfinished business" on style of care.

Institutional and Agency Issues

- There is less reimbursement or none for children's hospice and home care.
- High staff-intensity caring is required for children at home.
- Ongoing staff support is necessary.
- Children's services have immediate appeal to public.
- Special competencies are needed in pediatric care.
- How admission criteria may screen out children need to be assessed.
- Unusual bereavement needs of family members need to be assessed.

Adapted from Kuebler KK, Berry PH. End-of-life care. In: Kuebler KK, Berry PH, Heidrich DE, eds. *End-of-Life Care: Clinical Practice Guidelines*. Philadelphia: WB Saunders; 2002:25,[12] used with permission; and Children's Hospice International. http://www.chionline.org. Accessed February 23, 2005, prepared by Paul R. Brenner.[13]

during implementation of neonatal palliative care measures, while realizing the uniqueness of each situation.

Palliative Care Plans

Catlin and Carter[10] developed a palliative care protocol that has been disseminated widely since 2002. It is one of the only evidence-based plans available. Since the creation of this protocol, other dimensions of neonatal palliative care have been developed. For example, in 2007, the National Association of Neonatal Nurses (NANN) published a position statement on "NICU Nurse Involvement in Ethical Decisions Treatment of Critically Ill Newborns,"[14] and Rogers and colleagues[15] developed an educational program to address issues of moral distress in NICU nurses.

Advocacy for Support Services

Nurses can serve as advocates to ensure that the family is offered extensive support. Providing these services is crucial for the family unit to maintain a sense of wholeness during this challenging time. The following is taken from the 2012 NANN position statement on palliative care for newborns and infants.[16]

Appropriate family support services should be provided, including the following:

- Perinatal social workers, hospital chaplains, and clergy to provide emotional and spiritual support
- A child life specialist or family support specialist to support the infant's siblings
- A family advocate (a parent who has had a child in the NICU) to assist with navigating the NICU experience
- A lactation consultant to assist mothers who want to breastfeed their infant or donate breast milk at the end of life and to help mothers manage cessation of lactation at the end of life[17]

The nurse should not underestimate the impact that palliative and end of life care discussions can have on each member of the healthcare team during the transition through difficult clinical scenarios. The nurse can feel torn between spending quality time with a dying child and family and caring for other neonatal patients. The emotional strain associated with end of life and bereavement care not only affects a nurse's health but also can affect relationships at home and with coworkers.[18] In the past decade, more attention has been paid to the role of the nurse and the sense of moral distress that can exist when a nurse is providing care for infants who continue to decline clinically. Catlin and colleagues noted that the most commonly reported cause of nurses' distress was having to follow orders to support end of life patients with advanced technology when palliative or comfort care would be more humane.[19] Parents may sense the moral distress when the nurse is not receiving adequate peer support during the delivery of intensive care measures. It is vital that nurses have a forum to process their concerns within a confidential and professionally supported environment.

Debriefing sessions and clinical case reviews for difficult neonatal cases can be helpful. Team support can also come in the form of relief or "emotional rest" periods for the neonatal nurse; for example, a nurse who has experienced a recent neonatal end of life care case may benefit from having patients with more stable clinical trajectories for the next few patient care assignments. Jonas-Simpson and colleagues suggest that education and support in nursing practice could be enhanced by providing workshops and seminars on perinatal loss and bereavement care; incorporating discussions on supporting families, patients, colleagues, and oneself in bereavement care during unit orientation and ongoing education; debriefing after perinatal loss; and providing with a bereavement mentor for staff.[20]

New Trends

In 2003, the End-of-Life Nursing Education Consortium (ELNEC) developed a neonatal and pediatric version of the ELNEC curriculum. To date, 650 pediatric and neonatal nurses have received this education in the United States and abroad (http://www.aacn.nche.edu/elnec). More institutions are interested in neonatal-specific content to start their own palliative care teams. Despite support from the American Academy of Pediatrics and the World Health Organization for the provision of palliative care, there are still many barriers. Kain[21] identified these neonatal palliative care barriers as formal educational needs on the part of staff, a feeling of failure (especially by the physicians), difficulty in communicating bad news to the parents, and ethical conflicts among the team members. There is demonstrated evidence through the interest in ELNEC that nurses around the world wish to provide good palliative care as a standard part of neonatal care.

Summary of the Benefits of Palliative Care

Neonates who would benefit from excellent palliative care could die minutes, months, or years after birth, with a life-threatening anomaly or illness. The nurse is called on to focus on providing care when the prognosis is uncertain, and this may challenge existing healthcare system structures. The trajectory can be unpredictable, and the focus needs to be on providing excellent pain and symptom management while promoting developmental care of the infant, as well as maintaining adequate emotional, psychosocial, and spiritual support for the family. Families and professionals have the difficult task of helping the infant live as fully as possible with complete dignity and comfort while preparing for and accepting that the infant may not live a long time. This requires a committed interdisciplinary team with community linkages, as appropriate. Nurses new to palliative care should have the support of more senior nurses and staff because the first infant death experience can cause the nurse a considerable amount of anxiety and emotional distress.

Regardless of the length of life or the place where that life is lived, palliative care includes providing optimal symptom relief for the neonate, honoring the parents' wishes, providing ongoing support to parents and family, planning for the death, and honoring the life by creating memories of the life. The nurse should avoid phrases such as "withdraw care" or "nothing more can be done." There are always interventions that can be done to promote comfort during end of life care for infants with complex chronic conditions. These include supporting pain, managing secretions, minimizing sleep disturbances, treating agitation, and optimizing the time that can be spent peacefully with the family. Table 4.3 lists common medications used during the infant's end of life care. The use of a neonatal scale should continue during end of life care.[16] Supportive care should continue throughout the bedside postmortem care and incorporate options for obtaining mementos. In some regions, there are bereavement photography specialists who can assist with providing compassionately developed photographs of the deceased infant (see "Now I Lay Me Down to Sleep" at https://www.nowilaymedowntosleep.org/find-a-photog).

Neonatal End of Life Palliative Care Protocol*

The purpose of this protocol* of care is to educate professionals and enhance their preparation and support for a peaceful, pain-free, and family-centered death for dying newborns.

Planning for a Palliative Care Environment

To begin a palliative care program, one must realize that some institutions find it difficult to confront the issue of a dying child. So to begin to create a palliative care environment, there must be staff education and buy-in. This education must address cultural issues that affect caregiving. Ethical issues must be addressed either by the group creating the environment or by consultants who specialize in ethics.

Staff must treat the family as care partners, not as visitors. They must recognize that someone needs to be available 24/7 to address issues such as advance directives and symptom and pain management, both in the hospital and at home, if discharge is possible. There must be a mechanism to prepare the community for the child's entrance home or to hospice. This includes what to say to friends, relatives, and visitors.

Prenatal Discussion of Palliative Care

It is essential that fetal development and viability be discussed with all families, including those receiving assisted reproductive therapies, as part of prenatal care packages and classes. As the course of prenatal care progresses, pregnant women should be made aware that newborns in the very early gestational

---

* This protocol was published in Kenner C, Lott JW. *Neonatal Nursing Handbook*. St. Louis: Mosby; 2003:506-525. Adapted from Texas Children's Cancer Center–Texas Children's Hospital. *End-of-Life Care for Children*. Houston: Texas Cancer Council; 2000.[8]

Table 4.3 Palliative Care Medications for Neonatal Patients

Medications	Usual Dose	Special Considerations
For Pain		
Morphine	0.02–01 mg/kg IV q2–4h PRN 0.2–0.4 mg/kg PO q2–4h PRN 0.02–0.1 mg/kg/h	Opioid; medication of choice for pain management in palliative and end of life care May use in combination with benzodiazepine More frequent doses may be needed to ensure patient comfort
Fentanyl	1–3 mcg/kg IV or intranasal q1–2h PRN 1–3 mcg/kg/h	Fast onset and short-acting opioid Use injection form to administer intranasally; bioavailability is almost 90% Preferred in patients with renal failure
Methadone	0.05–0.2 mg/kg IV or PO q4–24h	Long-acting opioid Usual starting frequency is every 8–12 h scheduled Peak onset is delayed and may require breakthrough pain medication for 48 h after initiation or dose escalation
Acetaminophen	10–15 mg/kg PO q4–6h PRN 20 mg/kg PR q6h PRN 7.5–10 mg/kg IV q6h PRN	Analgesic; antipyretic May give IV form undiluted over 15 min
Oral sucrose 24%	<1 kg: 0.1 mL PO PRN 1–2 kg: 0.5 mL PO PRN >2 kg: 1–2mL PO PRN	Analgesic; may administer directly into mouth or apply on pacifier.
For Pain/Sedation		
Clonidine	1–3 mcg/kg PO q6–8h	Alpha agonist; has mild analgesic and sedating properties; may cause hypotension and bradycardia; avoid use of patch in neonates
For Sedation		
Midazolam	0.05–0.1 mg/kg IV q1h PRN 0.2 mg/kg sublingual or intranasal q1h PRN 1-2 mcg/kg/min	Very short-acting benzodiazepine Anticonvulsant, sedating, produces amnesia; rapidly penetrates the central nervous system During end of life care, more frequent doses may be needed to ensure patient comfort
Lorazepam	0.05–0.1 mg/kg IV or PO q2–4h PRN	Benzodiazepine Reduces anxiety and agitation; anticonvulsant Consider adding to opioids for sedation

(continued)

Table 4.3 (Continued)		
Medications	**Usual Dose**	**Special Considerations**
Diazepam	0.05–0.25 mg/kg PO or PR q4–12h	Long-acting benzodiazepine; peak onset is delayed and may require breakthrough with shorter acting benzodiazepine for 24–48 h after initiation or dose escalation
		Reduces anxiety and agitation; anticonvulsant
		Consider adding to opioids for sedation
For Secretions		
Glycopyrrolate	2–10 mcg/kg IV q6h 20–100 mcg/kg PO q6h	Decreases oral secretions through anticholinergic activity; increase slowly to effective dose; consider reducing dose if signs of tachycardia noted
Glycerin suppository	$\frac{1}{8} - \frac{1}{4}$ suppository PR q12–24h PRN	Osmotic laxative; consider using with opioids to reduce constipation

Adapted from Stevens B, Yamada J, Ohlsson S. Sucrose for analgesia in newborn infants undergoing painful procedures. *Cochrane Database Syst Rev.* 2004;3:CD001969;[22] and Walter-Nicolet E, Annequin D, Biran V, et al. Pain management in newborns: from prevention to treatment. *Pediatr Drugs.* 2010;12:353–365.[23]

periods of 22 to 24 weeks, and with birth weights of less than 500 grams, may not be responsive to resuscitation or applied neonatal intensive care.

Physician Considerations

The families need honest, straightforward language. They need to know their options, and it is essential that they understand what to expect. Usually the physician delivers this information, but the nurse is generally the one that can help the parents sort through feelings and grasp what they were told. If there is a sudden event, such as an unexpected premature or complicated birth, then the family's ability to comprehend and retain what is being said is limited. Reinforcement at a later time is advisable.

Family Considerations

Peer support from families that have experienced a similar infant illness or death may help the family cope. If the family finds out that the pregnancy is not viable, then it is up to the healthcare team to support the family's needs and to garner resources, such as other family members, spiritual counselors, and friends. Helping the family experience the normal parenting tasks, such as naming the baby, is very appropriate and helpful. This allows the family to gain some control, "parent," and build memories.

Transport Issues

It is best that mothers not be separated from their newborn infants. Transport is considered both traumatic and expensive, and if the newborn's condition is incompatible with prolonged life, then arrangements to stay in the local hospital may generally be preferred. It is best to avoid transferring dying newborns to Level III NICUs, if nothing more can be done there than at the local hospital. The local area is recognized as that location where parents have their support system, rapport with their established healthcare providers, a spiritual/religious community, and funeral availability.

The key to whatever decision is made, referral or not, requires good, clear communication with the family and between the two institutions. The family should not feel they are being sent away or given the wrong message by the nature of the transfer, or even return from a tertiary center once a referral is made if there is nothing to be done. The family needs a consistent message if trust is to be developed.

Which Newborns Should Receive Palliative Care?

Although many aspects of palliative care should be integrated into the care of all newborns, there are infants born for whom parents and healthcare professionals believe that palliative care is most appropriate. The following categories of newborns have experienced the transition from life-extending technological support to palliative care. The individual context of applying palliative care will require that each case, in each family, within each healthcare center, be explored individually. These newborn categories are provided for educational purposes and to engender discussion at the local institutional level.

- Newborns at the threshold of viability
- Newborns with complex or multiple congenital anomalies incompatible with prolonged life, for whom neonatal intensive care will not affect long-term outcome
- Newborns not responding to intensive care intervention, who are deteriorating despite all appropriate efforts, or in combination with a life-threatening acute event

Introducing the Palliative Care Model to Parents

Speaking to parents about palliative care is difficult. The following points may help physicians and nurse practitioners facilitate the process:

- Let the family know they will not be abandoned.
- Assist the family in obtaining all of the medical information that they want. Tell them that the entire medical team wishes the situation were different. Let them know you will support them every step of the way and that their infant is a valued and loved member of their family.
- Hold conversations in a quiet, private, and physically comfortable space.
- Give them your beeper number or telephone number to call you after they have digested the information and have more questions. Offer the ability to have a second opinion and/or an ethics consultation.
- Provide parents time to consult the local-regional center that works with children with special needs or their area pediatrician, who can provide information on projected abilities and disabilities.
- Offer to introduce them to parents who have been in a similar situation.

- When possible, use lay-person language to clarify medical terms and allow a great deal of time for parents to process the information.

- Avoid terms such as "withdrawal of treatment," referring to the stopping of life support, or "withdrawal of care," referring to the stopping of feedings or other supportive interventions. Specifically explain the exact treatment or care that is to be terminated so that the intention is clear.

- Use terms such as "change in care" or "change in treatment."

- Communicate and collaborate with parents at all times. Clarify mutually derived goals of care for the infant. Give as many choices as possible about how palliative care should be implemented for their infant. Inform the parents of improved access to the infant for holding, cuddling, kangaroo care, and breastfeeding. Developmental care approaches such as these promote the building of an infant-parent relationship.

- If the transition in care involves the removal of ventilatory support, explain that the use of ventilators is for the improvement of heart/lung conditions until cure, when cure is a likely outcome.

- Tell the parents that you cannot change the situation but you can support the infant's short life with comfort and dignity. Explain that discontinuing interventions that cause suffering is a brave and loving action to take for their infant.

- Validate the loss of the dreamed-for healthy infant but point out the good and memorable features the infant has. Help parents look past any deformities and work to alleviate any blame they may express.

- Encourage parents to be a family, as much as possible. Refer to the newborn by name. Assist them in planning what they would like to do while the infant is still alive.

- Encourage them to ask support persons to join them on the unit. Facilitate sibling visitation. Support siblings with child life specialists on staff.

- In daily conversation, avoid terms that express improvement, such as "good," "stable," or "better" in reference to the dying patient, so as not to confuse parents.

- Prepare the family for what may happen as the infant dies.

- Introduce families to the chaplain and social worker early in the process.

Optimal Environment for Neonatal Death

When the decision is made that a newborn infant may be close to death, there are several components to optimizing the care. These include the following:

- Compassionate, nonjudgmental, consistent staff for each infant, including physicians knowledgeable in palliative care. If consistent staff is not an option in a particular unit, then agreement on the plan of care is essential, with proposed revisions to care discussed with the whole team.

- Nurses and other healthcare staff educated in providing a meaningful experience for the family while caring for the family's psychosocial needs, including a period of time after the death.

- Parents who are educated in what to expect and who are encouraged to participate in, or even orchestrate, the dying process and environment of their infant in a manner they find meaningful.

- Staff and facility flexibility in responding to parental wishes, such as participation of siblings and other family members, and including wishes of parents and families who do not wish to be present.

- Institutional policies that allow staff flexibility to respond to parental wishes.

- Providing time to create memories, such as allowing parents to dress, diaper, and bathe their infant, feed the infant (if it is possible), take photos, and hold the infant in their arms. If they wish to take the infant outdoors to a peaceful and natural setting, that should be encouraged.

- Siblings should be made comfortable; they may wish to write letters or draw for the infant. Snacks should be available.

- Allowing the family to stay with the infant as long as they need to, including after death occurs.

- The process for treating the dying infant[10,24,25] is well described in the literature and by the various bereavement programs. Such processes include having one nurse assigned to be with the family, staying with the infant while parents take breaks, and collecting mementos that families may wish to take home (e.g., pictures or videos, handprints and footprints, and locks of hair).

- Parents should be assisted in making plans for a memorial service, burial, and so forth. Some parents might wish to carry or accompany the infant's body to the morgue or to the funeral home. Issues such as autopsy, cremation, burial, and who may transport the body should be discussed, especially if the parents are far from home and wish to transport the body to their home area for burial. In some states, hospitals may release a body to parents, after notifying the county department of vital statistics. The family must sign a form for removal of the body. The quality assurance department should be notified. Further discussion of autopsy and organ and tissue donation issues is included.

Location for Provision of Palliative Care

Location is not as important as the "mindset" of persons involved in end of life care. The attitude of staff, their desire to care for dying newborns and their families, their training in observation, support, and symptom management, and their knowledge of how to apply a bereavement protocol are more important than the physical location of the patient. Many agree that an active NICU may not be the optimal place for a dying newborn. Whether the infant is moved to a room off of the unit (e.g., a family room), moved to a general pediatrics ward, or kept on the postpartum floor, the best available physical space with privacy and comfort should be chosen.

The families need help to make the decision of how and where the infant is to be given care. If families take the infant home, coordination with the emergency medical services (EMS) personnel may be necessary to prevent undesired intervention. Parents need to be instructed not to call 911 because in some places emergency medical technicians are obligated to provide cardiopulmonary resuscitation (CPR). A letter describing the diagnosis, existence of in-hospital do-not-resuscitate (DNR) order, and hospice care plan for home, with the full expectation that the patient will die, should be provided to the parents, their primary physician, home-health agency or hospice, and perhaps the county EMS coordinator. Generally, hospice nurses are allowed to confirm a patient's death.

Ventilator Removal and Pain and Symptom Management

At times, cessation of certain technologic supports accompanies the provision of palliative care. The following information addresses (1) how to prepare the family, staff, and facility for discontinuation of ventilator support, and (2) the process of removing the ventilator in a manner that minimizes discomfort for the infant and the family. The latter includes who will be present at the time of extubation. A plan must be worked out with the family about what medications and support will be given to alleviate pain and suffering and what they can expect the dying process to be like for their baby. Consideration of developmentally supportive care, attuned to ambient light and noise as well as comfort measures, are important. These should incorporate cultural considerations.

Mementos can be obtained by nurses, such as a lock of hair, handprints or footprints in plaster, and photos and/or videotapes of the family together, if this is culturally appropriate. If the infant has serious anomalies, photos of hands, ears, lips, and feet can be provided. Ear prints and lip prints are possible. Some parents have indicated that mementos of a newborn who died are not acceptable in their culture.

When Death Does Not Occur After Cessation of Aggressive Support

A private room in the hospital is recommended, with nurses trained in palliative care. If the expected time for expiration passes and death does not occur, the infant could be discharged to home for ongoing palliative care services. The parents, NICU staff, and hospice staff should meet to make plans for home care, including the investigation of what services are offered and what insurance will cover. Continued palliative care or hospice services with home nursing care is essential, including the possibility of ventilator removal at home.

If the infant is to go home, a procedure for dispensing outpatient medications should be in place. All needed drugs and directions for use should be sent along with the infant so that the parents do not have to go to a pharmacy to fill prescriptions. Identifying and communicating with a community healthcare provider who will continue with the infant's home care needs is essential.

Some families and healthcare providers think that dying newborns should be fed, and if they are unable to suck, should be tube-fed. Others think that artificial feeding is inappropriate. Withholding feedings is an ethical dilemma for many health professionals and families and needs careful consideration.[26] Recent research indicates that feeding can be burdensome and that an overload of fluids can impede respirations.[27] In all cases, infants should receive care to keep their mouth and lips moist. Drops of sucrose water have been found to be a comfort agent, if the infant can swallow, and they may be absorbed through the buccal membrane.

Parents who feel they cannot take the infant home should be assisted to find hospice care placement.

Discussion of Organ and Tissue Procurement and Autopsy

At some point in the course of care, organ and tissue donation and autopsy will need to be discussed. Before discussion with families, the regional organ donation center should be contacted to determine whether a particular infant qualifies as a potential donor. In some areas, only corneas or heart valves are valuable in an infant weighing less than 10 pounds, but in different locations, other organs (e.g., heart) or tissues may be appropriate. It is important to know whether a newborn has no potential donor use and to communicate this respectfully. Parents often desire the ability to give this gift and may be doubly hurt if they wish to help others and are turned down.

The person who discusses organ and tissue procurement must be specially trained. Although the physician usually initiates this, a nurse, chaplain, or representative from donor services may conduct the conversation with tact and compassion. The provider should be aware of cultural, traditional, or religious values that would preclude organ donation for a specific family because many cultures and religions would consider this desecration of the dead infant.

Suggestions Concerning Autopsy

Requests for autopsies are not required in all states but may be considered appropriate in many instances of infant death. If the medical examiner or coroner is involved in the case, laws may require autopsy. Some providers feel that asking for an autopsy is important to potentially provide parents with some answers regarding their infant's illness and death. The placenta may also be used for testing to provide information. In the discussion, parents may wish to know all or some of the following:

- Autopsy does not cause any pain or suffering to the infant; it is done only after death.
- The body is handled with the ultimate respect.
- Some insurance companies pay for a physician-ordered autopsy.
- Final results are returned in approximately 6 to 8 weeks, at which time the primary physician can meet with the parents, conduct a telephone conference, or communicate by letter to discuss the results.

Family Care: Cultural, Spiritual, and Practical Family Needs

The hospital social worker is an essential component of supportive palliative care. Families may immediately need financial assistance, access to transportation, and a place to stay.

Practical Considerations

Parents of multiples, in which some lived and one died, will need special attention to validate their bereavement, as well as to support their love for their living children.

Time should be permitted for the parents to contact the needed author-ity in their culture and to plan any necessary ceremony, some of which may require special permission; for example, use of incense.

Cultural Sensitivity

These support needs should be anticipated and provided, as much as possible:

- When using a translator, simple words and phrases should be used so that the translator can convey the exact message. It is most appropriate to use hospital-trained and certified translators to ensure accuracy.
- Whenever possible, written materials should be given in the family's pri-mary language, in an easy-to-read format that is culturally and linguistically appropriate for the family.
- Culturally sensitive grief counseling and contact with a support group of other parents who have been through this are helpful.

Family Follow-Up Care

Families who have experienced a neonatal death will likely leave the facility in a shocked state. Families can best be served by the following:

- Establishing contact with a social worker, chaplain, or grief counselor before discharge
- Receiving an information packet as described and a date for a follow-up discussion with the attending physician (which may be in conjunction with autopsy results)
- Notifying the family's obstetrician of the death, no matter how long after delivery it occurred
- Arranging a home visit by one of the staff or a public health nurse within a few days
- Making phone calls weekly, then monthly, then at 6-month intervals, if parents agree
- Providing contact on significant days, such Mother's Day, the infant's due date, or the anniversary of the infant's death.
- Inviting the family to a group memorial service held by the hospital for those who have lost pregnancies or infants in the past year
- Keeping in mind that subsequent pregnancy may be difficult and offering support at that time, including genetic counseling if indicated
- Keeping snapshots and mementos on the unit, if parents do not wish to take them at the time, because some parents may reconsider later

Ongoing Staff Support

The work of providing end of life care for newborns and their families is very intense. Staff needing support are not limited to the nursing staff and include physicians and all healthcare and ancillary personnel who have interacted with the infant or family. Suggested support includes the following:

- Facilitated meetings of the multidisciplinary team during the process, especially if some of the team members are reluctant to change to this mode of care
- Debriefings after every infant's death and after any critical incident

- Meetings or counseling sessions that are part of regular work hours and not held on voluntary or unpaid time
- Moral support for the nurses and physicians directly caring for the dying newborn provided by peers as well as the unit director, other neonatologists, chaplain, and nursing house supervisor
- Nursing staff scheduling that is flexible and allows for overtime to continue with the family or to orient another nurse to take over
- If they wish, notifying the primary nurse and physician if they are not present at the actual time of the infant's death
- With permission of the parents, allowing the primary nurse and physician to attend the funeral, if desired, and to take time off afterward, if needed

Acknowledgments

We would like to acknowledge Beth Seyda and her family for sharing their journey and experiences with the death of their beloved son, Dylan. We would also like to acknowledge Dr. Margarita Bidegain, Associate Professor of Pediatrics, Duke Children's Neonatology Division, for her support and encouragement throughout the editing of this chapter.

References

1. Caitlin A. Transition from curative efforts to purely palliative care for neonates: Does physiology matter? *Adv Neonatal Care.* 2011;11(3):216-222.

2. Ahern K. What neonatal intensive care nurses need to know about neonatal palliative care. *Adv Neonatal Care.* 2013;13(2):108-114.

3. Moro TT, Kavanaugh K, Savage TA, et al. Parent decision making for life support decisions for extremely premature infants: from the prenatal through end-of-life period. *J Perinat Neonatal Nurs.* 2011;25(1): 52-60.

4. Wigert H, Dellenmark MB, Bry K. Strengths and weaknesses of parent-staff communication in the NICU: a survey assessment. *BMC Pediatr.* 2013;13:71.

5. Wool C. Clinician confidence and comfort in providing perinatal palliative care. *J Obstet Gynecol Neonat Nurs.* 2013;42(1):48-58.

6. Institute for Patient- and Family-Centered Care. 2013; http://www.ipfcc.org/. Accessed April 24, 2015.

7. Hockenberry MJ, Wilson D. *Wong's Nursing Care of Infants and Children.* 8th ed. St. Louis: Mosby; 2006.

8. Texas Children's Cancer Center–Texas Children's Hospital. *End-of-Life Care for Children.* Houston: Texas Cancer Council; 2000.

9. Catlin A. Extremely long hospitalizations of newborns in the United States: data, descriptions, dilemmas. *J Perinatol.* 2006;26:742-748.

10. Catlin A, Carter B. Creation of a neonatal end-of-life palliative care protocol. *J Perinatol.* 2002;22:184-195.

11. Anand KJS. Pharmacological approaches to the management of pain in the neonatal intensive care unit. *J Perinatol.* 2007;27:S4-S11.

12. Kuebler KK, Berry PH. End-of-life care. In: Kuebler KK, Berry PH, Heidrich DE (eds.) *End-of-Life Care: Clinical Practice Guidelines*. Philadelphia: W.B. Saunders; 2002:25.

13. Children's Hospice International. http://www.chionline.org. Accessed February 23, 2005.

14. National Association of Neonatal Nurses (NANN). NANN position statement 3015: NICU nurse involvement in ethical decisions (treatment of critically ill newborns). *Adv Neonatal Care*. 2007;7(5)267-268.

15. Rogers S, Babgi A, Gomez C. Educational interventions in end-of-life care. Part I: an educational intervention responding to the moral distress of NICU nurses provided by an ethics consultation team. *Adv Neonatal Care*. 2008;8(1):56-65.

16. National Association of Neonatal Nurses. Palliative care for newborns and infants: position statement #3051. September 2010; http://www.nann. org/uploads/files/Palliative_Care-final2-in_new_template_01-07-11.pdf. Accessed April 24, 2015.

17. Moore DB, Catlin A. Lactation suppression: forgotten aspect of care for the mother of a dying child. *Pediatric Nurs*. 2003;29(5):383-384.

18. Zhang W, Lane BS. Promoting neonatal staff nurses' comfort and involvement in end of life and bereavement care. *Nurs Res Pract*. 2013;2013:365329.

19. Catlin A, Volat D, Hadley MA, et al. Conscientious objection: a potential neonatal nursing response to care orders that cause suffering at the end of life? Study of a concept. *Neonat Netw*. 2008;27(2):101-108.

20. Jonas-Simpson C, Pilkington FB, MacDonald C, McMahon E. Nurses' experiences of grieving when there is a perinatal death. *Sage Open*. 2013;3(2):21582 44013486116.

21. Kain VJ. Palliative care delivery in the NICU: what barriers do neonatal nurses face? *Neonat Netw*. 2006;25(6):387-392.

22. Stevens B, Yamada J, Ohlsson S. Sucrose for analgesia in newborn infants undergoing painful procedures. *Cochrane Database Syst Rev*. 2004;3:CD001969.

23. Walter-Nicolet E, Annequin D, Biran V, et al. Pain management in newborns: from prevention to treatment. *Pediatr Drugs*. 2010;12:353-365.

24. Oosterwal G. *Caring for People from Different Cultures: Communicating across Cultural Boundaries*. Portland, OR: Providence Health System; 2003.

25. American Hospital Association (AHA). A patient's bill of rights. http:// www.injuredworker.org/Library/Patient_Bill_of_Rights.htm. Accessed April 7, 2015.

26. McHaffie HE, Fowlie PW. Withdrawing and withholding treatment: comments on new guidelines. *Arch Dis Child*. 1998;79:1-2.

27. Craig F, Goldman A. Home management of the dying NICU patient. *Semin Neonatol*. 2003;8:177-183.

Additional Neonatal Palliative Care Resources

Academy of Neonatal Nursing: http://www.academyonline.org/

Association of Women's Health, Obstetric and Neonatal Nurses: http://www. academyonline.org/

Centering Corporation (perinatal grief books and literature): http://www.centering.org/

Certification in Perinatal Loss Care (CPLC): http://www.nbchpn.org/

End-of-Life Nursing Education Consortium (ELNEC) Pediatric Palliative Care: http://www.aacn.nche.edu/elnec/about/pediatric-palliative-care

Hochberg T. Moments held—photographing perinatal loss. *Lancet.* 2011;16:1310-todd@toddhochberg.com

Institute for Patient- and Family-Centered Care: http://www.ipfcc.org/

National Association of Neonatal Nurses: http://www.nann.org/

Resolve Through Sharing (RTS) Bereavement Training: Perinatal Death: http://www.bereavementservices.org/resolve-through-sharing/conferences-and-workshops/perinatal-death-training

Unspoken Grief: http://unspokengrief.com/

Chapter 5

Pediatric Care

*Transitioning Goals of Care in
the Emergency Department,
Intensive Care Unit, and in Between*

Barbara Jones, Marcia Levetown, and Melody Brown Hellsten

Palliative care is comprehensive, transdisciplinary care focused on promoting the maximal quality of life for patients living with a life-threatening illness and their families.[1] Palliative care is as applicable in the emergency department (ED) and in the intensive care unit (ICU) setting[2] as it is in the home.[3] This is a critically important issue for children who die because most childhood deaths occur in an ICU setting.[4]

Epidemiology of Pediatric Death

Approximately 48,000 children die annually in the United States.[5] Infants (children younger than 1 year), who account for close to 50% of childhood deaths, die primarily of congenital defects and prematurity; however, sudden infant death syndrome (SIDS) and trauma (including unintentional injury and homicide) account for 13% of infant deaths.[6] For children aged 1 to 24 years, 65% of deaths are the result of trauma, whereas the remaining 35% are the result of cancer, congenital anomalies, infection, and metabolic defects.[6] Traumatic injury and unexpected overwhelming illness occurring in previously healthy children usually call for initial resuscitative measures provided in ED and ICU settings; many of these children may unavoidably die there, too. In fact, 20% of childhood deaths are declared in the ED each year, whereas 4.6% of pediatric ICU and 10% to 20% of trauma ICU admissions end in death, together accounting for 40% to 90% of childhood deaths.[7] Consideration of palliative care issues must therefore be a part of the care plan for critically ill or injured children at admission to the ED and the pediatric intensive care unit (PICU), as well as at discharge if the child survives.[2] Bereavement care for families, including siblings, is a critical but often neglected need when pediatric death occurs in acute care settings.[2]

Palliative Care Considerations in the Emergency Department and Intensive Care Unit

Acute Unexpected Illness or Injury

Children experiencing a life-threatening event can present to the ED having been transported either by their parents or by emergency medical system (EMS) providers after a potentially dramatic on-site resuscitation effort. The initial scene in the ED is often one of controlled chaos, with all personnel attending to the assessment and stabilization of the child. Some of these children are trauma victims, benefiting from a thorough assessment, rapid intervention, and pain control before a prognosis can be determined. For the child arriving in full arrest, the overwhelmingly likely outcome is death, whether in the ED or in the ICU a few days later.[8] In the absence of severe trauma, intoxication, or congenital heart disease, primary cardiac causes of arrest among children are exceedingly rare. Thus, if cardiac arrest has occurred, the child is either irreversibly dying of multi-organ failure or has sustained prolonged hypoxemia; neither of these underlying causes of arrest is amenable to resuscitation with intact survival. The unlikelihood of a good outcome following resuscitation from cardiac arrest must be addressed in the care of these children and their families.

Needs of Parents of Suddenly Ill or Injured Children in the Emergency Department

Assigning a professional to guide the parents from the moment of their arrival can facilitate communication, even given the severe time pressures of the ED.[9] This professional should greet the parents by name, introduce himself or herself, and provide a card with his or her name and contact information. The family should be apprised of the child's situation, and the child should be referred to by name.[9] This guide should also address parents' practical needs, such as offering a blanket or water and assisting in gathering the family's supporters. An interpreter should be summoned immediately, if needed.

Especially in the ED, parents of acutely injured children prefer to be given timely, accurate, and consistent information that is easy to understand.[9] Information given should be responsive to family members' questions and concerns. Extended family members or friends can often help the parents sort through the information and help them know what to ask. Although "information" emphasizes content, the nuances of "communication," or the process by which information is exchanged, are important as well. All family members of critically ill or dying children need to feel respected and valued. Grief and worry under these extraordinarily stressful circumstances can be totally debilitating and incapacitating. This is the context in which parents are often asked to make decisions that, when worded poorly, imply choices between life and death; it may also be the context of their experience of the last hours with their child.

Parents need to be given the opportunity to be with their child, even when he or she is undergoing cardiopulmonary resuscitation or other invasive procedures. Recent studies validate that parents can be present without disrupting the care process and that their bereavement outcomes are enhanced when given this opportunity.[10] However, physicians and nurses express a wide range of opinions and comfort levels with family presence during resuscitation. Written policies and staff education are needed to address family presence.

Gradual disclosure of the child's condition enables the parents to better absorb the information that the child is likely to or has died. Although it is generally recommended that the attending physician be responsible for the disclosure of death, a study of parent preference found that parents preferred someone who is knowledgeable and compassionate and that they were unconcerned about the individual's title. The child's usual care providers should be notified of the death as well, particularly the primary care pediatrician, who should be alerted to closely monitor the well-being of siblings in the aftermath of death.

When a child dies in the ED, his or her parents may prefer to be invited to be with their child's body in a private setting, for as long as they need to stay; they often wish to bathe and rock or hold the child's body. This may be difficult to accommodate in the ED but can have a tremendously beneficial effect on the family's recovery.[9] Ideally, the body will be cleaned up and fresh linens will be placed around it, with any disfiguring or gaping wounds covered, before inviting the parents to hold the child. Having the opportunity to speak with a chaplain and social worker at this time is often greatly appreciated. Even more important, parents need to understand the sequence of events, have their questions answered, and have supportive witnesses to their and their child's experience. Parents often want a physical memento of their child, such as a lock of hair, a mold of the child's hand, or their child's hospital bracelet and clothing. Some families appreciate being assured that the child's body will not be left alone until the funeral director or coroner comes to retrieve it.

Children With Chronic Life-Threatening Conditions in the Intensive Care Unit

Unfortunately, even children with chronic illnesses and anticipated deaths most often die in the ICU.[4] This is less often a result of the circumstances of the death than of a lack of advance care planning, largely related to an uncertain prognosis.[11]

Ideally, the patient and family facing a chronic, progressive, and ultimately fatal illness would be provided information gradually and recurrently, in an outpatient setting. That information would be tailored to the child's particular condition and the family's value system, related by a long-standing primary care physician.[1] Families need to understand the anticipated trajectory of the child's chronic condition and its associated symptoms; the interventions available for life extension and their likely outcomes, benefits, and burdens; the likely causes of death; the fact that symptoms can and will be controlled, regardless of the goals of care; and, most important, that that they will not be abandoned.[1,12,13] Preemptive discussions, when the child is stable, can help the child contribute to the discussion and aid in developing the family's preferences for end of life and a coordinated plan of care. Parents have stated that the opportunity for advance care planning provides them with comfort and assurance that their child received proper care.[12] Nurses often play a leading role in initiating such discussions. Table 5.1 provides suggestions on how to begin this discussion during a stable period of a life-threatening condition. Additional advice is found in an article by Mack and Wolfe.[14]

Table 5.1 Communicating With Children and Families About Integrating Palliative Care	
Beginning the conversation	"What is your understanding of what is ahead for your child?"
	"Would it be helpful to talk about how his or her disease may affect him or her in the months and years ahead?"
	"As you think about what is ahead for your child, what would you like to talk about with me? What information can I give you that would be helpful to you?"
Introducing the possibility of death	"I am hoping that we will be able to control the disease, but I am worried that this time we may not be successful."
	"Although we do not know for certain what will happen for your child, I do not expect that your child will live a long and healthy life. Most children with this disease eventually die because of the disease."
	"I have been noticing that your child seems to be sick more and more often. I have been hoping that we would be able to make him or her better, but I am worried that his or her illness has become more difficult to control and that soon we will not be able to help him or her to get over these illnesses. If that is the case, he or she could die of his or her disease."
Eliciting goals of care	"As you think about your child's illness, what are your hopes?"
	"As you think about your child's illness, what are your worries?"
	"As you think about your child's illness, what is most important to you right now?"
	"You mentioned that what is most important to you is that your child be cured of his or her disease. I am hoping for that too. But I would also like to know more about your hopes and goals for your child's care if the time comes when a cure is not possible."
Introducing palliation	"Although I hope that we can control your child's disease for as long as possible, at the same time I am hoping that he or she feels as good as possible each day."
	"Although it is unlikely that this treatment will cure your child's disease, it may help him or her to feel better and possibly to live longer."
Talking about what to expect	"Would it be helpful to talk about what to expect as your child's illness gets worse?"
	"Although we cannot predict exactly what will happen to your child, most children with this disease eventually have [difficulty breathing]. If that happens to your child, our goal will be to help him or her feel as comfortable as possible. We can use medications to help control his or her discomfort."

(continued)

Table 5.1 (Continued)	
Talking to children	"What are you looking forward to most of all?"
	"Is there anything that is worrying you or making you feel afraid?"
	"Is there anything about how you are feeling that is making you feel worried or afraid?"

Reprinted with permission from Mack JW, Wolfe J. Early integration of pediatric palliative care: for some children, palliative care starts at diagnosis. *Curr Opin Pediatr.* 2006;18(1):10-14.[14]

Continuity and Coordination of Care Needs

Parents need to know what care venues are available to them in the community and how to access them to avoid recurrent, no-longer-beneficial ICU admissions in the setting of a chronic, life-limiting condition.[1,15] Children with terminal conditions and their families often want spiritual consultation and guidance because it is very hard to understand why so tragic a thing as a child's death has to occur.[16] If end of life care is properly provided, fewer children with chronic, life-threatening conditions will die in the ICU and instead will die in a setting that they or their family members prefer.[11]

Therapies that are not consistent with the child's and family's goals or that will not work given the child's condition should not be offered to children who have experienced chronic, progressive illness. In addition, misperceptions about the effectiveness of cardiopulmonary resuscitation in life-threatening conditions must be proactively addressed. Proposals to forgo medical interventions should be presented with justifications and as a recommendation, not a choice, for the family to make alone. Importantly, when suggesting what should no longer be done, describe what will be added or maintained to enhance the child's and family's quality of life. One suggested phrase that captures the essence of intensified caring with new goals is: "We will help your child live to his/her fullest to the very last moment, regardless of when that is. His/Her comfort and yours are our top priority."

Child Participation in Decision-Making

Most state advance directive laws do not specifically mention children. Although there is no legal mandate to address the issues of prognosis or potential future medical interventions with chronically ill children, the intent of advance directives applies equally to children with decision-making capacity as to adults. Developing advance directives for children ensures that the wrenching decision-making process is well considered and that the resulting care plan is enacted when the child's inevitable deterioration occurs, preventing an unwelcome ICU admission. Families state that advance care planning for their children provides them peace and hope,[11] enabling them to decide based on the children's best interests and to include the child's perspective, when possible.[17] It is recommended that the discussion be a longitudinal process, initiated early after the onset or discovery of life-threatening illness, maintained throughout the course of a child's illness, and documented in written form.

Advance care planning can prevent ED and ICU deaths for children who prefer to die at home; however, discussions of advance care planning frequently happen late in the disease or illness trajectory. Durall and colleagues[18] found that while 92% of providers believed that advance care planning should happen early or during moments of stability, 60% indicated that those conversations were more likely to occur when death was imminent or a crisis was occurring. Whenever possible, the knowing child (who may be as young as 3 years if he or she has been chronically ill) should have a voice in the discussion of the goals of medical intervention. Children and adolescents can and should be involved in end of life planning, and there are resources such as *My Wishes* and *Voicing My Choices* available to assist healthcare providers and family members in having these conversations with patients.[17,19] When the child cannot be involved, the effect of parental guilt ("I can't let my child go—it would mean I failed as a parent") and family suffering on the decision-making process should be frankly discussed.[20] Reminding parents of their obligation to decide in their child's best interests and reassuring them that letting go is a loving decision can be helpful.

In states with out-of-hospital do-not-resuscitate (DNR) laws, ensuring that these forms are appropriately executed (if the family chooses this option), that the medical home physician and local EMS are involved or at least notified, and that hospice care is arranged can be very helpful to families. These activities increase the likelihood that the child will die at home, where most children and adults would prefer to die.[11]

In the ICU or ED, when the chronically ill child is not responding to stabilization or resuscitative efforts, the parents are often asked, "Do you want us to do 'everything'?" This question does not fully encompass the possible benefits and burdens and probable outcomes of potential interventions. From the parent's perspective, there is no reasonable answer to this question but "Yes!" However, for informed consent to occur, the goals and the understanding of likely outcomes must be discussed and aligned before proceeding. To the physician, "everything" too often means everything to prolong survival, regardless of the quality of life. For parents, other goals generally take precedence.[11] If the child's condition is stabilized and symptoms are aggressively controlled, more rational decision-making can take place.

Table 5.2 provides suggested phraseology to ensure clear communication and to prevent perceptions of abandonment.

Death Related to Chronic, Progressive Illness

Issues Relevant to Emergency Department and Intensive Care Unit Personnel

Although communicating news regarding the terminal phase of chronic disease is difficult and stressful for everyone, being uninformed of the severity of the situation is even more stressful for patients and families. One of the most common complaints of patients and families is the lack of accurate and

Table 5.2 Methods of Communicating Sensitive Healthcare Information and Perceptions of Communication

Usual Method of Communicating Message	How the Usual Communication May Be Perceived	Alternative Method of Communicating Message
"Do you want us to do CPR?"	"CPR would work if you would allow us to do it."	"Tell me what you know about CPR. CPR is most helpful for patients who are relatively healthy, and even then, only 1 of 3 patients survives. Many of Lisa's organs are not working. As you know, she is getting dialysis to clean her blood like her kidneys would have, a breathing machine for her lungs, and medicine to keep her blood pressure up. If her heart were to stop, it would not be because there is a problem with her heart (it is fine), but it would be because she is dying. All of our hearts stop when we die. So pumping on her heart, or "doing CPR" will not make her better. On the other hand, while I would recommend not doing CPR, I am not recommending stopping any other treatment she is receiving at this time. There is still a chance that she may get better. Let's hope for the best, but also plan for the worst. We will need to keep a close watch on her and keep you up to date on how she is doing. Do you have any questions?" "Let's talk again later today so I can update you. Is there anyone else I need to talk to?"
"Let's stop heroic treatment."	"We will provide less than optimal care" (What is heroic about performing invasive, painful, costly, nonbeneficial care?)	"At this time, I think the most heroic thing we can do is to understand how sick Jamal is and stop treatments that are not working for him. I think we should do all we can to ensure his comfort and yours, make sure there are no missed opportunities, and ensure we properly celebrate his life. I will follow your lead on this. Some ideas that have helped other families include getting him home with help for you if you wish, or you may choose to have his friends and your family come here instead and have a party; you can bring his clothes so that he will look like himself, bring in his music or a photo album and relive some of your best memories of him, make a mold of his hand so that you will always have his hand to hold, or anything else that would be a proper celebration of his life."

(continued)

Table 5.2 (Continued)

Usual Method of Communicating Message	How the Usual Communication May Be Perceived	Alternative Method of Communicating Message
"Let's stop aggressive treatment."	"We will not be attentive to his needs, including symptom distress and need for comfort"	"We will do all we can to ensure he is as comfortable as possible."
"Aiesha has failed the treatment."	"The patient is the cause of the problem"	"We have tried all the proven treatments and even some experimental ones for Aiesha. Unfortunately, we did not get the results we had hoped for. I wish it were different!"
"We are recommending withdrawal of care for Marisa."	"We are going to abandon her and you."	"Marisa is too ill to get better. We need to refocus our efforts on making the most of the time she has left."
"There is nothing more we can do for Adam."	"We will allow him to suffer, we do not care about him, we only care about fighting the disease."	"We need to change the goals of our care for Adam. At this point we clearly cannot cure him, but that does not mean we can't help him and your family."
"Johnny is not strong enough to keep going."	"Johnny is weak."	"Johnny is a strong boy and he has fought hard with us to beat his disease. Unfortunately, as much as we wish we could, we cannot save Johnny. At this point, we are hurting him rather than helping, giving him side effects, and keeping him from being at home or taking a trip, or whatever he really wants to do with the time he has left."
"We will make it so Thuy does not suffer."	"We are going to kill Thuy."	"We will do everything we can to make Thuy comfortable."
"We need to stop active treatment for Dwayne."	"We will not take care of him at all."	"The goal of curing Dwayne's disease, despite the best efforts of a lot of smart and hard-working people, is no longer possible. We are so sorry and wish that that were different! I have cared for many children who are as sick as your son. It is very hard on all of us, especially you, his parents and family, when the treatments do not work as we had hoped. Many parents like you have agreed to stop efforts to cure when they are not working, as difficult as that is. Would you like me to put you in touch with some of the other parents who have been through this too?"

(continued)

104

Table 5.2 (Continued)

Usual Method of Communicating Message	How the Usual Communication May Be Perceived	Alternative Method of Communicating Message
"Do you want us to stop Bobby's treatment?"	"You are the final arbiter of your child's death."	"Bobby is lucky to have such excellent, loving, and selfless parents. I know this is hard; we will get through it together. I am glad you agree with our recommendations to change the goals of care to better meet Bobby's needs. I will let my team know what we have decided."
"I am glad you agree. Will you sign Juan's do-not-resuscitate order?"	"You are signing his death warrant."	"There is no surgery, no medicine, and all the love you clearly feel for Juan will not make him better, he is just too sick. I wish it were different." (Silence) "I will change his orders to make sure he only gets tests and treatments that can help him now."

CPR, cardiopulmonary resuscitation.

Reprinted with permission from Levetown M. Communicating with children and families: from everyday interactions to skill in conveying distressing information. *Pediatrics.* 2008;121(5)e1441 -e1460.[21]

clearly communicated information.[1,2] Done well, disclosure of the prognosis associated with a chronic condition often provides confirmation for families of what was already suspected, frequently resulting in relief and reduction of anxiety.[1]

Suggestions for discussing a poor prognosis in a way that is sensitive to the needs of the child and family, as well as the medical caregivers, are found in Box 5.1.

Patient and Family Needs in the Intensive Care Unit

Entering an ICU or ED is a frightening experience for both the child and family, regardless of the presenting problem, prognosis, or treatment plan. The environment of care significantly affects the ability of families to cope, particularly if the child dies.[2] ED and critical care providers must strive to remember that the experience is new and often terrifying for children and families. Interventions to alleviate this type of suffering can improve the immediate experience of the child and the long-term outcomes for the parent.

High levels of post-traumatic stress disorder (PTSD) have been demonstrated among family members of ICU patients[23]; providing even minimal information regarding how an ICU works, identifying the personnel involved and their functions, and teaching families how to access information have a dramatically beneficial effect. A simple explanatory brochure can lower ICU family PTSD rates by 50%. In addition, support and honest communication are an important intervention.

Box 5.1 Having Difficult Discussions

1. Provide a "warning shot" or an introductory sentence before presenting the distressing information: "I am sorry that I have some bad news to tell you."

2. Provide an opportunity for supportive friends or family to be present when the information is shared: "Would you like to call someone to be with you when we talk?"

3. Tell the news in a private setting, with the physician, nurse, and social worker present. Bring the family (generally parents without the child first, depending on relationships and preferences) to a private conference room, rather than speaking to them in the waiting room or the hall. Bring tissues. If appropriate and desired by the family, assist them in telling their children (patient and siblings) afterward.

4. Sit down near the family, not across a table. Do not stand. Children and families want to be on an even plane with their caregivers. Look the family members in the eye to engender trust unless this is culturally undesirable. Ask them to tell you about their child and about the things that give him or her pleasure. Ask how much they want to know about his or her medical condition and prognosis. Ask them what they understand is happening. Clarify misconceptions, particularly about the cause of the problem, and attempt to assuage any guilt that may derive from having an inherited or developmental problem ("You did not wish for your child to have this") or from trauma or other causes. Then, let them know this news is difficult for you as well. Nurses can help guide the physician to present the truth in a jargon-free manner that is consistent with the family's educational level, sophistication, and stated desire for knowledge. Ask the family to explain what they understood was said. Clarify misconceptions. Then, solicit additional questions.

5. Be unhurried. If there is only a limited time available for the physician, let the family know: "I'm sorry the doctor only has 15 minutes now, but I will stay with you and answer any questions I can, and the doctor will be back later this afternoon to answer anything I can't and to update you." Don't look at your watch. Have the charge nurse or another nurse care for your patients while you sit with the family. Remind the other team members to give their beepers to someone else during the family meeting, when possible; otherwise, switch the beepers to vibrate mode.

6. Ideally, members of the multidisciplinary team participate as full members during the family conference.[12] The bedside nurse, chaplain, and social worker benefit from hearing the physician-family interaction. They can solicit questions, clarify misconceptions during the meeting, and after the physician leaves, address other facets of the patient's situation that the conversation evokes. Team members can also give the physician feedback regarding his or her communication with the patient and family, such as words they did not understand, and can help the physician address any unresolved issues at the next meeting. This technique requires interdisciplinary respect and cooperation, which are essential to

(continued)

Box 5.1 (Continued)

successful, comprehensive end of life care; it prevents divisive misunderstandings between disciplines.

7. Bring trainees to the family meeting. This allows the assigned nursing or medical student and resident to learn by directly observing the interdisciplinary critical care team, as well as the patient and family responses. It informs trainees so that unnecessary and often damaging miscommunications do not occur. Trainees often get lost in the minutiae of the patient's laboratory values and vital signs and may unwittingly provide contradictory information to the family. However, do not overwhelm the family with white coats—have trainees take turns attending family meetings.

8. Be specific. The physician should present the options, include a description of life-sustaining treatments, the child's current status, the chance of survival, the probability of full recovery (and the probability of significant disability), and the possible effects of the child's long-term survival on the family.

Adapted from Edlynn ES, Derrington S, Morgan H, et al. Developing a pediatric palliative care service in a large urban hospital: challenges, lessons, and successes. *J Palliat Med*. 2013;16(4):3 42-348[12]; and Hain R, Heckford E, McCulloch R. Paediatric palliative medicine in the UK: past, present, future. *Arch Dis Child*. 2012;97(4):381-384.[22]

Needs of the Child in the Intensive Care Unit

In addition to being included in advance care planning and having meticulous symptom control, ill children also benefit from having a member of the healthcare team attend specifically to their emotional needs. Ideally, the critical care unit has a social worker or child life specialist who is immediately accessible and able to provide critical assessment, support, distraction, and intervention for children who are alert and can participate.

Compassionate, Effective, Consistent Bidirectional Communication

Compassionate, effective, consistent bidirectional communication with the family and the patient is critical to providing care and preventing suffering. Research on the needs and priorities of families whose child died in the ICU reveals that effective and compassionate communication is of primary importance. Parents need to retain the role of caregiver and protector of their child and to function within the context of the family unit, regardless of circumstance. Recent studies have demonstrated that the time of first discussions between medical staff and parents and definitive decision-making in the pediatric ICU can vary from immediate to 19 days, with large variations between decision-making and actual withdrawal of life-sustaining treatment.[24,25] Communication and collaboration should occur with families at the earliest possible point to enhance decision-making and family-centered care.

Strategies for Improving Team Communication

Nurses are often key professionals when it comes to communication with families in the ICU. Being at the bedside, nurses often get to know well the families and their concerns, values, and priorities and can enable the correct approach to best meet the needs of each family. Participation of the bedside nurse in daily rounds and in family meetings improves continuity of care and consistency of information and communication. The information that nurses gather from patients and parents at the bedside is critically important to the entire team for understanding what the patient and family already know, what questions they have, and what further explanations or discussions are needed. In addition, excellent communication between nurses at shift change is needed about what the family has been told and what they seem to understand. Parents often call at night to check on their children and get confused by conflicting messages. Strategies and tools, such as primary nursing assignments and communication logs or a "goals of care" worksheet, can improve overall communication and quality of care.

Effective Communication With Families

In complex environments like the ED and ICU, it is critical that members of the healthcare team also communicate effectively with each other, in order to avoid confusion and resulting distress. Communication in highly technical and emotional circumstances can be difficult. The family's willingness to acknowledge or accept a potential prognosis, physician bias regarding the goals of care, the management of and tolerance for uncertainty, and the emotions of the healthcare professional or family can create obstacles to open, honest communication regarding the child's condition and prognosis. Positive communication styles include being receptive to patient and family cues, demonstrating genuine concern, moral responsibility, and a caring and dedicated presence. Many clinicians try to "shield" parents from bad news because they are reluctant to "take away hope." However, research by Mack and colleagues [26] has demonstrated that what parents define as hope differs from caregivers' perceptions. Parents hope for honest information that allows them to make the best decisions for and with their child and to have the capacity to ready themselves for the inevitable with the support of their loved ones.

End of Life Family Conferences

End of life family conferences have been identified as an important communication tool in the pediatric ICU and constitute the keystone around which excellent end of life care can be built. Ideally all members of the interdisciplinary pediatric team will participate in the family conference.

End of life family conferences are formal, structured meetings between physicians, staff, and family members. Family conferences require honest, clear information about the patient's condition and treatment and willingness on the part of physicians to listen and respond to family members and to address their concern and emotions. Shared decision-making based on clarity of prognosis, goals, and a clear plan of care allows the healthcare team and family to engage in continuous, compassionate, and technically proficient attention to the child's needs until death occurs.

Medical Decision-Making

Clarity of facts and ethical principles among family and staff enables good medical decision-making. Despite the benefits of formal family meetings, communication of difficult information is a process, not an event. Respect between the healthcare team and family is essential for the family to trust the guidance of the team and participate in decision-making regarding preferences for care. This can be accomplished by encouraging patients and families to share their story, concerns, and preferences for care, listening without interruption, and clarifying areas of misunderstanding. Nonverbal cues such as eye contact, humility, and respect go a long way toward building trust. The team should then allow families to arrive at decisions in a time frame that is comfortable for them.

Families of ICU patients have an increased risk of posttraumatic stress symptoms; some develop full-blown PTSD.[23] The risk was increased among families who felt that insufficient time was available for receiving information, who felt that information was incomplete or difficult to understand, who participated in end of life decision-making, and whose loved one died during the hospitalization.[23]

Time-Limited Trials

The patient's progress over the course of ICU care should be continuously reviewed with the patient and family. Monitoring whether the patient is progressing along the hoped-for improvement trajectory or whether he or she is deteriorating provides real-time information to facilitate care planning and decision-making. Frequent updates, attentive communication about the child's condition, and reasonable medical interventions help families avoid burdensome and unhelpful medical interventions and allows preparation for death as a likely outcome.[2]

Recommendations for the next clinical step should be presented based on the team's experience with similar patients, the goals and values of the patient and family, and the observations of patient and family members during the meeting and the hospitalization overall. The benefits and burdens (including prolongation of suffering) of each potential care plan, the potential reversibility or irreversibility of the conditions being treated, the time frame for reevaluation, the projected future quality of life, and the comfort measures available if the ICU interventions are curtailed or discontinued must be explained to the family in a manner they can understand.

When discussing the choice to forego no-longer-beneficial medical interventions, the topics of current burdens of therapy and the probability of the hoped-for benefits must be clearly explained. Reassure the family that if ICU interventions are discontinued, the child will continue to receive attentive care for symptom relief; describe the procedures to be undertaken, including the opportunities to observe important customs and rituals and the visitation allowances. The benefits of stopping ED or ICU treatments can be presented as limiting the harm to and suffering of the child and enabling the loving presence of the family. When the option is inaccurately presented as "stop-ping care," it is, not surprisingly, usually rejected. This shorthand phraseology is sometimes perceived as cruel and callous; patients and families fear aban-donment above all else. Word choice is critical. Some hospitals have begun to use "Allow Natural Death, or "AND," as a replacement or adjunct to DNR discussions. Although there is no consensus on the use of AND, it does pro-vide another way to facilitate compassionate discussions with families.[27]

End of Life Decision-Making

In most clinical situations, the justification to forgo disease-directed medical intervention in ICUs involves physician assessment of poor prognosis for sur-vival rather than patient quality-of-life considerations. Parents, however, make their decisions based on the child's quality of life, degree of pain and suffering, likelihood of improvement, and physician's recommendations, as well as the child's "will to live," knowledge of other deaths, and perceptions of the child's best interests.[28] Reassessing the goals of treatment only when the child is dying may deprive the patient and family of earlier choices to limit suffering, rather than extending the duration of life. Children and their families often have preferences regarding the value of medical interventions during palliative care. Their opinions are not knowable by the medical team a priori; they must be actively solicited.

Consideration of Suffering and Future Quality of Life

Surrogates' (or parents') duties are to act on the child's wishes and in his or her best interests. Healthcare practitioners should work closely with families to make the best decisions regarding continuation or termination of ICU interventions. Thus, overriding any requests to terminate ICU inter-ventions must be done with significant forethought and analysis. In addition, the motivation for requests to continue ICU interventions in the face of an extremely small likelihood of survival or a significantly poor quality of life must be explored fully. Guilt, fear, and loss issues, in particular, should be examined.

A child's or surrogates' requests to stop ICU interventions must be taken seriously in order to determine current sources of suffering, eliminating them where possible, reducing them, or changing the goals of care. The request may indeed signal the time to focus on maximizing comfort, regardless of effect on life expectancy.[2] Suffering experienced by the child must play a much more prominent role in the decision-making process if maximal comfort and support are to be attained for a higher proportion of dying pediatric patients.[11] ICU physicians and nurses must be educated on ethical principles in medical practice, particularly on autonomy, beneficence, nonmaleficence, and the construct of benefits versus burdens in making and guiding decisions. Personal biases regarding quality versus quantity of life, fears of litigation, and economic motivations must not play any role in decisions regarding the withdrawal of ICU interventions.

Within practical limitations, the patient's comfort should be the primary determinant in end of life care. In several studies, vasopressors were withheld first, then oxygen, and then mechanical ventilation. However, oxygen supplementation and extubation may be preferred and more comfortable, potentially providing the opportunity for a last goodbye. In addition, withholding antibiotics and allowing the peaceful death associated with sepsis, without a trip to the ICU, may be the most humane option available for some children. In other cases, forgoing nutrition may ease nausea, and forgoing hydration may decrease the discomfort of renal failure or congestive heart failure.[29] Obviously, much depends on the child's symptoms, the clinical situation, and the child's and family's values and preferences. Effecting a philosophical change among medical decision-makers to proactively solicit children's and families' perspectives may be accomplished by educational intervention, although it is likely that cultural changes within institutions and protocol-driven practice may have more promise.

Forgoing No-Longer-Beneficial Intensive Care Unit Interventions

Review of the Patient Care Plan

After it has been determined that the child's and family's primary goal is no longer to prolong of life, because either the child's suffering is too great or the child will die no matter what is done, the care plan must be reviewed in detail. The most probable mechanisms of death must be determined. Possible symptoms can then be anticipated and a care plan created to address proactively the child's comfort. Developmentally appropriate explanations about the possible course of events should be given to the child and family, unless they refuse this information. It is unwise to predict an exact time of death, but approximations (with significant margin for error—e.g., minutes to hours, hours to days, days to weeks) are helpful for the family to arrange for the child's other loved ones and friends to visit before or be present at death.[2]

All interventions that interfere with comfort should be discontinued in favor of interventions aimed at promoting maximal comfort, function, and quality of life.[2] For example, laboratory tests are not designed to enhance comfort. Sometimes in clinical practice, laboratory parameters, such as platelet counts, are monitored to "prevent" symptoms (such as bleeding) from arising. However, it is less intrusive to monitor the patient for clinical bleeding and treat if and when it arises. Medications that do not enhance comfort, including antibiotics, should be considered for discontinuation. Even feeding and intravenous fluids may interfere with comfort if the child has pulmonary edema, heart failure, or renal failure; a decrease in or cessation of these therapies may enhance the child's comfort.[2] Removal of no-longer-needed devices, including monitoring equipment, should also be considered.

Forgoing No-Longer-Beneficial Critical Care Interventions

Forgoing mechanical ventilation precedes most ICU deaths, allowing patients a more peaceful death.[2] Although a common phenomenon, many critical care practitioners are uncomfortable with this decision. Initiating a meeting of those involved in the care of the patient to review the choice and hear concerns, as well as to guide the care, is very helpful in minimizing distrust and maintaining staff cohesion. Protocols that outline the ethical principles underlying such choices are helpful in guiding decision-making and management of the extubation by critical care physicians and nurses.

When a family elects to forgo treatments in anticipation of death, visitation restrictions and many of the usual rules should be reconsidered. Opportunities to hold the child and even invitations to family members to climb in bed with the child should be facilitated. Letting the family bathe the child and dress him or her in clothing of the child's or family's choice is often helpful. Other requests should be honored, if at all possible.

Engaging in family-centered rituals before forgoing critical care interventions is important, allowing unhurried family time while the child is still alive. As the family is approaching readiness for extubation, they should be reminded about what changes they are likely to see in the child, making this difficult time easier. ("He may turn blue; we will treat this with morphine and oxygen, if he looks uncomfortable. He may not breathe at all or may breathe comfortably for some time. His breathing may be noisy, because his brain is not controlling his throat's soft tissues. I do not know how long he will live, but I expect it will be on the order of (minutes, hours, days). I will stay with you until he is comfortable.") Positive thoughts about extubation are important to share as well. ("This will be the first time you see your daughter's beautiful face, without tape and a tube interfering"; "I am giving you back your son as a child, not as a patient"; "You may be able to hear his voice for the first time in a while," depending on the age and circumstances of the child.)

Extubation Technique

There is no single correct way to discontinue mechanical ventilation.[2] Although adult care practitioners most often wean the patient's ventilator settings and leave a tracheal tube in place, it is not clear that this is what families prefer. Pediatric practitioners more often remove the tracheal tube. Although some practitioners premedicate before changing ventilator settings, others wait to see how the patient responds.[30] It is best to understand the parents' hopes for the final minutes to hours of their child's life, to educate them about the potential likelihood of achieving them, and then to make every attempt to honor their wishes. The goal of preventing any discomfort at all calls for preemptive sedation,[30] conflicting with a goal of a final goodbye. These considerations should be discussed in advance.

Transfer to Alternative Care Settings

When children are acknowledged to be dying, it is common for extended family and loved ones to gather to support each other. Sometimes they may desire to perform rituals that are difficult to accommodate in the ICU setting. Thus, consideration of transferring to an alternate care setting may be helpful, even if it is only for a few hours.

If the child is anticipated to live for a few days after critical care interventions are discontinued, referral to hospice in the home care setting may be an option, particularly in the United Kingdom.[31] Usually, a 1- to 2-day stay in the hospital to ensure "stability" and to provide family and hospice caregiver teaching is needed. Alternatively, if the child will have significant distress in his or her final days, or if the child and family prefer to stay in the hospital, admission to the floor, or preferably a palliative care unit, may be the best plan. With the increase of pediatric palliative care programs in the United States and elsewhere, it is becoming more possible for providers to refer or collaborate with the palliative care service. An agreement to transfer out of the ICU must usually be predicated by an agreement to terminate the ventilator within hours of transfer.

Aggressive Symptom Management in the Emergency Department and Intensive Care Unit

Aggressive symptom control is a high priority for parents of children who die.[2] When critical care technologies are forgone, the most common symptom-distress risks are dyspnea, pain, and seizures.[2] Thus, meticulous care at the time of ventilator withdrawal, including the continuous presence of the physician or nurse, and protocols for symptom management are key to the effective prevention or immediate management of symptom distress.[2] When attended to by a skilled interdisciplinary team that focuses on these issues as primary concerns, symptoms are usually successfully prevented or rapidly mitigated. It is helpful to most families to affirm their decision and to explain the possible events in advance of their occurrence.

Pain

Pain in the ED may be acute, related to trauma, procedures, or infections, or may be related to exacerbations of chronic, painful conditions among children with complex medical illnesses. Age-appropriate assessment tools and evidence-based pain management approaches, including distraction, local anesthetics, oral analgesics, and sedation, as appropriate, should be employed to minimize the child's pain.[32]

Assessment and management of pain in the ICU setting are confounded by the likely use of sedative and paralytic agents if the child is intubated. A number of pain assessment scales are validated for the pediatric ICU patient, including the Premature Infant Pain Profile (PIPP), children's pain checklist, and FLACC (Face, Legs, Activities, Cry, and Consolability) and COMFORT scales.[33] The Individualized Numeric Rating Scale can be used with children with severe cognitive impairment.[1]

The occurrence of pain is not well documented in the terminally ill pediatric ICU patient, but suspicion of pain must remain high, and presumptive treatment should occur if indications of pain are present. When possible, pain needs to be categorized not only by severity but also by character (burning, gnawing, throbbing, sharp, crampy), location and radiation, duration, continuous or intermittent nature, and precipitating and relieving factors. The quality and timing of the pain suggest the etiology of the pain and dictate the most efficacious treatment. This ideal is very difficult to achieve in young or developmentally disabled children and in sedated or intubated patients. An empirical judgment of the etiology and physiology of the pain often dictates the choice of intervention in the ICU setting.

Medications should be titrated to pain control using acetaminophen or nonsteroidal antiinflammatory around-the-clock pain relief (unless contraindicated), in addition to opioids for more severe pain, opioids and local anesthetics for procedure-related pain, and "adjuvant" analgesics for neuropathic pain. "As needed" or PRN opioid doses should be ordered for the alleviation of breakthrough pain. Medications should also be available for the expected side effects of opioids, such as nausea, pruritus, urinary retention, and somnolence (when it is undesirable). Changing the specific opioid used[34] may also be considered for the management of refractory opioid-induced side effects when the child's expected survival is longer. Alternative routes of pain relief, such as epidurals for children who are excessively somnolent or who become delirious with systemically administered opioids, may be of benefit in some cases.[1]

Constipation

Constipation is common in the ICU. Risk factors for constipation in the ICU include immobility, dehydration, and use of opioid, sedative, and paralytic medications. Nurses should consistently document bowel movement patterns and report lack of bowel movement greater than 2 days. Adjuvant stool softeners and laxatives should be initiated for any nonambulatory, sedated, or intubated patient.

Dyspnea

When the choice is to discontinue or to not initiate mechanical ventilation, scrupulous attention to the assessment and management of dyspnea must be explained and promised to the child (if capable of participating) and the family, and the promise must be realized. The idea that there may be a tradeoff between relief of dyspnea and sedation, or even a slightly earlier death, must also be broached, concerns addressed, and preferences elicited. In the few studies reviewing duration of survival related to the administration of morphine during withdrawal of mechanical ventilation, however, patients of all ages actually survive longer when liberal doses of morphine are used to ease the dyspnea.[2] Most families opt for enhanced comfort, even in the face of a potentially foreshortened survival. However, patients occasionally are much less distressed than anticipated and are able to enjoy a few hours or even days with carefully titrated opioids.[34]

Dyspnea is a symptom that is even more distressing than pain to experience or witness. Behavioral correlates of the sensation of dyspnea observed in ICU patients are (in decreasing order): tachypnea and tachycardia, a fearful facial expression, use of accessory breathing muscles, paradoxical (diaphragmatic) breathing, and nasal alar flaring. Dyspnea can be difficult to control and requires intensive hands-on management and reassessment. Several nonpharmacologic approaches can be helpful,[35] such as limiting fluid intake, sitting the child upright, having a parent or other close family member or friend present, saying soothing words, and touching the child. In addition, having a small fan blow air across the child's face has been helpful in the hospice setting.

Regardless of the protocol used, it is imperative that the child be continuously observed; the dose should be rapidly and aggressively escalated until relief is achieved. The "correct" dose is established by titration to clinical effect; there is no maximal dose of a pure opioid. Documentation should reflect dosing in response to distress and, optimally, will also note its resolution in response to treatment.[34,36]

Thorough suctioning of endotracheal tubes before extubation of mechanically ventilated children is helpful in preventing dyspnea and "death rattle."

Palliative Sedation

Occasionally, a technique known as palliative (or sometimes "total") sedation is necessary to control refractory symptoms, most often pain, dyspnea, and intractable seizures. Within the palliative care community, palliative sedation has become a generally accepted option for refractory symptom management in adults. There are published articles for its use in children as well.[37,38] Palliative sedation is the extension of the tenet that, above all, the healthcare provider's duty is to relieve suffering. The intention is not to bring about the demise of the child (as in the case of physician-assisted suicide and euthanasia),[39] but rather to control the symptom, even at risk of death (principle of double effect).[34,40]

Regardless of the philosophical underpinnings that lead to the practice, palliative sedation is widely regarded in palliative care circles as the only humane solution to an otherwise uncontrollable and severely distressing problem. It is only undertaken after all other attempts at symptom control by an expert have failed to bring comfort. Full agreement of the child (when possible and usually accomplished in advance care planning discussions) and the family is required. Explanations of the inability to reverse the underlying disease process must precede this decision.[41]

Rituals and Activities That Celebrate the Child's Life

Most communication about forgoing "life support" concentrates on what will be stopped and not what will be enhanced or added.[12,15] Although we cannot help the child live longer, we can help parents properly celebrate the wonder of this child and the child's relationships, value, and impact she or he has had on the world.[2,42] Suggestions for accomplishing this include the following:

- Inviting friends and extended family to visit with the family and child
- Bringing the child's own clothing and dressing him or her in it after a bath (the parent may choose to do this or ask to have the nurse do this)

- Removing no-longer-needed medical devices ("to make him your child again, and not a patient")
- Making a three-dimensional plaster hand mold ("so you will always have your child's hand to hold")
- Bringing in photo albums to remember the good times that were had
- Bringing a camera or video to commemorate the celebration
- Offering families the opportunity to invite members of the family's congregation or others to provide spiritual support and guidance
- Bringing the child's favorite music, toys, videos, or other means of demonstrating the child's uniqueness
- Performing cultural, religious, or family rituals as appropriate

Families have unique, individualized ways of acknowledging their child. One family may bring balloons and a sheet cake; another may choose to apply a teen's makeup and favorite cologne; a third might play videos of the teen's victorious football game. Easy access to a rocking chair or couch for the parent to hold the child (no matter how large) is helpful. Offer unlimited coffee, water, juice and soft drinks.

Notification of Death in the Emergency Department or Intensive Care Unit When Parents Are Not Present

Unless there are extremely extenuating circumstances, even if the death is expected, most experts strongly encourage that the notification of death be done in person ("Mrs. Smith, I am afraid I have some bad news. Could you come in to discuss it?"). Empathy can be more easily expressed in person by sitting close to the parents and siblings at the time of the discussion, perhaps even giving the bereaved a hug or shedding a genuine tear.[2] These small tokens of warmth and understanding help the family to know that the medical team cared about the child as a person. Additionally, insistence that the family come in allows them to see the dead child's body, facilitating the acceptance of the death and allowing the family to participate in important rituals, such as bathing the child's body, sometimes assisting in the removal of equipment, or sitting vigil as some cultures require. These activities result in improved bereavement outcomes for the parents, as well as the siblings.

Autopsy and Organ Donation

One of the most common complaints of bereaved families is that they still, even years later, do not understand the cause of their child's death. Most of the time this is because shock or poor communication prevented their integration of the information. However, sometimes the cause of death was not known to the healthcare providers; in still other cases, the physician is incorrect in his or her assessment. In fact, major unexpected findings related to death occurred in 28% of the autopsies in a recent pediatric study. Among 100 consecutive autopsies, these investigators found new information that had the potential to further clarify the causes of a child's death (53% of cases); inform the future reproductive choices of either the parents (10%) or siblings (8%); affect siblings' future healthcare (6%); or contribute to patient care quality control (36%) or publishable knowledge (7%).[43] For these reasons, autopsy should be encouraged. Burial or cremation removes this opportunity.

Autopsies can be tailored to the needs of the family. Even the coroner's cases are not total body autopsies—they are limited to determining the cause of death. Most often, there is minimal disfigurement and an open-casket ceremony can still be performed if desired. Moreover, in elective autopsies, parents can choose to limit the autopsy to the organ of interest. It is possible to take needle biopsies rather than to remove whole organs, if preferred, and a request can also be made to replace all organs back in their natural locations after the autopsy is performed. Many locales do not charge the family for the autopsy. There is generally no more than a 24-hour delay in removing the body to the funeral home if an autopsy is performed.

Many parents of organ donors want follow-up information on the organ recipients' well-being.[44,45]

Post-Death Conference

One of the most frequently recommended ways to provide needed bereavement support for families of patients who died in the ICU or ED is the post-death conference.[2] Especially in sudden, unanticipated deaths, families cannot absorb new information about how and why the child died. It takes several weeks to begin to think more clearly; at that point, feelings of despair arise as the questions pour in. Parents often erroneously feel they were told nothing and can become angry about not understanding what happened. In addition, if an autopsy was performed, families may request a face-to-face appointment with the treating physician to explain the autopsy findings in understandable terms. This explanation can provide the bereaved family with a profound sense of peace by affirming the cause of death and the irreversibility of the problems or by determining a cause of death that was unknown ante mortem.

The post-death conference has even been found to improve adaptation to loss. It enables monitoring of the family's grieving process and provides the opportunity for referral to counseling, if needed, for pathological grief reactions. In the absence of a face-to-face session, families consenting to an autopsy often complain that they had no follow-up and express anger and suspicion about the autopsy motivations. This post-death conference is also helpful for families who did not consent to autopsy, to answer their inevitable questions. Referrals can be made for families needing counseling or other assistance.

Summary and Recommendations for Implementation

Improved end of life care begins with more highly focused attention on the individual child and his or her preferences and values. Pediatric and neonatal ICU and ED practitioners are the caregivers for most children who die; they must have expertise in palliative care. Infants die primarily of congenital defects, prematurity, and SIDS. Children older than 1 year of age die primarily from trauma, thus predisposing them to die in the ED or ICU settings. The principles of palliative care must be applied to all children, even those who die in the ED or ICU. Our challenge, as practitioners of pediatric emergency and critical care medicine, is to provide each of these children a "good death" and their families a more peaceful bereavement. This can be achieved by attention to the child's and family's perspectives and goals, communication within the team and with the child and his or her loved ones, dedication to the meticulous prevention and management of symptoms, particularly during procedures—the most common source of discomfort in ill children—and effective bereavement follow-up.

References

1. Klick JC, Hauer J. Pediatric palliative care. *Curr Probl Pediatr Adolesc Health Care*. 2010;40(6):120-151.

2. Truog RD, Campbell ML, Curtis JR, et al. Recommendations for end-of-life care in the intensive care unit: a consensus statement by the American College of Critical Care Medicine. *Crit Care Med*. 2008;36(3):953-963.

3. Vollenbroich R, Duroux A, Grasser M, et al. Effectiveness of a pediatric palliative home care team as experienced by parents and health care professionals. *J Palliat Med*. 2012;15(3):294-300.

4. Fontana MS, Farrell C, Gauvin F, et al. Modes of death in pediatrics: differences in the ethical approach in neonatal and pediatric patients. *J Pediatr*. 2013;162(6):1107-1111.

5. Kochanek KD, Kirmeyer SE, Martin JA, et al. Annual summary of vital statistics: 2009. *Pediatrics*. 2012;129(2):338-348.

6. Murphy SL, Xu JQ, Kochanek KD. Deaths: final data for 2010. *Natl Vital Stat Rep*. 2013;61(4):1-117.

7. Sands R, Manning JC, Vyas H, Rashid A. Characteristics of deaths in paediatric intensive care: a 10-year study. *Nurs Crit Care*. 2009;14(5):235-240.

8. Berg MD, Schexnayder SM, Chameides L, et al. Pediatric basic life support: 2010 American Heart Association guidelines for cardiopulmonary resuscitation and emergency cardiovascular care. *Pediatrics*. 2010;126(5):e1345-e1360.

9. DeVader TE, Albrecht R, Reiter M. Initiating palliative care in the emergency department. *J Emerg Med*. 2012;43(5):803-810.

10. Tinsley C, Hill JB, Shah J, et al. Experience of families during cardiopulmonary resuscitation in a pediatric intensive care unit. *Pediatrics*. 2008;122(4):e799-e804.

11. Dussel V, Kreicbergs U, Hilden JM, et al. Looking beyond where children die: determinants and effects of planning a child's location of death. *J Pain Symptom Manage*. 2009;37(1):33-43.

12. Robert R, Zhukovsky DS, Mauricio R, et al. Bereaved parents' perspectives on pediatric palliative care. *J Social Work End Life Palliat Care*. 2012;8(4):316-338.

13. Edlynn ES, Derrington S, Morgan H, et al. Developing a pediatric palliative care service in a large urban hospital: challenges, lessons, and successes. *J Palliat Med*. 2013;16(4):342-348.

14. Mack JW, Wolfe J. Early integration of pediatric palliative care: for some children, palliative care starts at diagnosis. *Curr Opin Pediatr*. 2006;18(1):10-14.

15. Rogers SK, Gomez CF, Carpenter P, et al. Quality of life for children with life-limiting and life-threatening illnesses: description and evaluation of a regional, collaborative model for pediatric palliative care. *Am J Hospice Palliat Med*. 2011;28(3):161-170.

16. Hexem KR, Mollen CJ, Carroll K, et al. How parents of children receiving pediatric palliative care use religion, spirituality, or life philosophy in tough times. *J Palliat Med*. 2011;14(1):39-44.

17. Wiener L, Zadeh S, Battles H, et al. Allowing adolescents and young adults to plan their end-of-life care. *Pediatrics*. 2012;130(5):897-905.

18. Durall A, Zurakowski D, Wolfe J. Barriers to conducting advance care discussions for children with life-threatening conditions. *Pediatrics*. 2012;129(4):e975-e982.

19. Aging with Dignity; Five Wishes. Voicing my choices. 2012; www.agingwithdignity.org. Accessed April 9, 2015.

20. Sharman M, Meert KL, Sarnaik AP. What influences parents' decisions to limit or withdraw life support?*. *Pediatr Crit Care Med*. 2005;6(5):513-518.

21. Levetown M. Communicating with children and families: from everyday interactions to skill in conveying distressing information. *Pediatrics*. 2008;121(5)e1441-e1460.

22. Hain R, Heckford E, McCulloch R. Paediatric palliative medicine in the UK: past, present, future. *Arch Dis Child*. 2012;97(4):381-384.

23. Kross EK, Engelberg RA, Gries CJ, et al. ICU care associated with symptoms of depression and posttraumatic stress disorder among family members of patients who die in the ICU. *Chest J*. 2011;139(4):795-801.

24. Oberender F, Tibballs J. Withdrawal of life-support in paediatric intensive care: a study of time intervals between discussion, decision and death. *BMC Pediatr*. 2011;11(1):39.

25. Shore PM, Huang R, Roy L, et al. Development of a bedside tool to predict time to death after withdrawal of life-sustaining therapies in infants and children*. *Pediatr Crit Care Med*. 2012;13(4):415-422.

26. Mack JW, Wolfe J, Cook EF, et al. Hope and prognostic disclosure. *J Clin Oncol*. 2007;25(35):5636-5642.

27. Jones BL, Parker-Raley J, Higgerson R, et al. Finding the right words: using the terms Allow Natural Death (AND) and Do Not Resuscitate (DNR) in pediatric palliative care. *J Healthcare Qual*. 2008;30(5):55-63.

28. McGraw SA, Truog RD, Solomon MZ, et al. "I was able to still be her mom"— parenting at end of life in the pediatric intensive care unit. *Pediatr Crit Care Med*. 2012;13(6):e350-e356.

29. Diekema DS, Botkin JR; Committee on Bioethics. Forgoing medically provided nutrition and hydration in children. *Pediatrics*. 2009;124(2):813-822.

30. Billings JA. Humane terminal extubation reconsidered: the role for preemptive analgesia and sedation. *Crit Care Med*. 2012;40(2):625-630.

31. Gupta N, Harrop E, Lapwood S, Shefler A. Journey from pediatric intensive care to palliative care. *J Palliat Med.* 2013;16(4):397-401.

32. Fein JA, Zempsky WT, Cravero JP, et al. Relief of pain and anxiety in pediatric patients in emergency medical systems. *Pediatrics.* 2012;130(5):e1391-e1405.

33. Zempsky WT. Optimizing the management of peripheral venous access pain in children: evidence, impact, and implementation. *Pediatrics.* 2008;122(Suppl 3):S121-S124.

34. Shaw TM. Pediatric palliative pain and symptom management. *Pediatr Ann.* 2012;41(8):329.

35. Quill TE, Lo B, Brock DW, Meisel A. Last-resort options for palliative sedation. *Ann Intern Med.* 2009;151(6):421-424.

36. Chidambaran V. Pediatric acute and surgical pain management: recent advances and future perspectives. *Int Anesthesiol Clin.* 2012;50(4):66-82.

37. Anghelescu DL, Hamilton H, Faughnan LG, et al. Pediatric palliative sedation therapy with propofol: recommendations based on experience in children with terminal cancer. *J Palliat Med.* 2012;15(10):1082-1090.

38. Morgan C, FitzGerald M, Hoehn K, Weidner N. 872: Pediatric palliative sedation and end of life care. *Crit Care Med.* 2012;40(12):1-328.

39. Lloyd-Williams M, Morton J, Peters S. The end-of-life care experiences of relatives of brain dead intensive care patients. *J Pain Symptom Manage.* 2009;37(4):659-664.

40. Wolfe J, Hinds PS, Sourkes BM. *Textbook of Interdisciplinary Pediatric Palliative Care.* Philadelphia: Elsevier/Saunders; 2011.

41. Anghelescu DL. Pediatric palliative sedation therapy with propofol: recommendations based on experience in children with terminal cancer. *J Palliat Med.* 2012;15(10):1082-1090.

42. Yang SC. Assessment and quantification of Taiwanese children's views of a good death. *Omega (Westport).* 2012;66(1):17-37.

43. Heller KS, Solomon MZ. Continuity of care and caring: what matters to parents of children with life-threatening conditions. *J Pediatr Nurs.* 2005;20(5):335-346.

44. Corr CA, Coolican MB. Understanding bereavement, grief, and mourning: implications for donation and transplant professionals. *Prog Transplant.* 2010;20(2):169-177.

45. Siminoff LA, Traino HM, Gordon N. Determinants of family consent to tissue donation. *J Trauma.* 2010;69(4):956.

Chapter 6

Grief and Bereavement in Pediatric Palliative Care

Rana Limbo and Betty Davies

"Effective and compassionate care for children with life-threatening conditions and their families is an integral and important part of care from diagnosis through death and bereavement."[1] This guiding principle, one of seven put forth by the Institute of Medicine report on the status of palliative and end of life care for children and their families, emphasizes that care continues for the family following the child's death. Although medical science has contributed significantly to the treatment of children with life-limiting illnesses or conditions, children still die from cancer, cardiac disease, respiratory conditions, genetic conditions, and more. Moreover, thousands of neonates die each year and thousands more children of all ages, particularly toddlers and adolescents, die as a result of trauma. Regardless of the cause, the death of a child is a tragedy, an incomparable life event that has an impact on all family members, friends of the family, and the community in which the family lives. A child's death also affects the physicians, nurses, social workers, and other healthcare personnel who provide care for the dying child.

Grief as a Process

Death is a part of each individual life, something we all must face, though we resist even the thought of our own mortality. The hoped-for pattern is that we experience deaths of others that are easier in earlier life, for us to build the skills to aid us with the more difficult deaths in later life. The death of one's child, though, sits outside of that hoped-for pattern. The grief associated with a child's death begins even before the actual death event, as the child's parents and other family members anticipate the death and experience the child's dying, and their grief continues long past the child's death. Many parents feel they never "recover" from the death of their child. They may resume daily activities, adjust to life without their child's presence, and find new pleasures in life, but many parents remain vulnerable and feel that they are not the same people they were before the child's death.[2-4]

Types of Grief

Anticipatory Grief

Anticipatory grief often occurs in advance of an expected loss. Rando[5] indicates that anticipatory grief entails grieving not just for future losses but also for losses that have already occurred and for current losses. It may be associated with the losses of expectations for a "normal" life that are associated with a particular diagnosis, with acute and chronic illness, or with death. Anticipatory grief occurs while the ill child is still alive, and this allows for hope. This is a subtle difference that makes anticipatory grief unique and helps account for what parents often describe as an "emotional roller coaster," particularly for parents of children with long-term chronic illness. Their experience of witnessing the child's physical deterioration and worsening of symptoms, interspersed with remissions, "good" days, and seeming progress toward health, lays fertile ground for emotional ups and downs and hope for the child's recovery. Over time, however, the focus of hope changes, and nurses can play a critical role in facilitating the expression of that hope. Initially, parents of children with cancer, for example, focus their hope on the possibility of cure. Each exacerbation chips away at the hope for the child's full recovery, and family members hope for longer remissions. Eventually, they hope their child will be able to live until he reaches a particular milestone, such as graduation, a special birthday, or the next holiday. As the child's condition worsens, parents may hope that their wish to care for their child at home will be possible and that their child will not suffer at the end. Hope is life sustaining; healthcare providers should support family members in their hope, refraining from crushing hope with overdoses of facts. In response to a mother's proclamation that her child will overcome a serious illness, the nurse can empathize, "I certainly do hope so." The death is anticipated, but it has not occurred, and in the parents' eyes, there is a chance, no matter how small, that it might not occur:

> My son has been to the PICU three times. At his first transfer to the PICU, my sorrow was beyond description. At that time, I thought I would never see him again. But my son has fought against his cancer every time. Whenever he came back to the ward from the PICU ... I remember recently that day was 3 days before his 13th birthday ... it was so amazing and I prayed thanks to God for allowing me to hope for his life again.

Although painful, anticipatory grieving does present an opportunity for families to begin to think about their future without the child. It can help family members begin to face the existential questions that arise when a child is dying. It can help families begin the process of reorganizing their fractured lives. Anticipatory grieving can also take its toll, especially when the child's illness endures. Rando[6] interviewed parents whose child had died from cancer and suggests there is an optimal length of anticipatory grief of 6 to 18 months. A shorter time did not give parents enough time to prepare for the loss, and a longer period had a debilitating effect on them.

Disenfranchised Grief

Disenfranchised grief acknowledges the social context of grief. It refers to the grief that persons experience when they incur a loss that is not or cannot be openly acknowledged, publicly mourned, or socially supported.[7,8] Those at risk include, for example, classmates, teammates, teachers, coaches, school bus drivers, crossing guards, or past boyfriends or girlfriends of the child or adolescent who died—those whose relationship with the now-deceased child or adolescent is not regarded as significant. Also feeling disenfranchised are those grieving a terminated pregnancy or a neonatal death for which the significance of these losses may not even be acknowledged or, if it is, such comments as, "You can try again" reflect insensitive misunderstanding of the parents' grief. Families of children with serious cognitive or physical limitations, from progressive neurodegenerative illnesses, for example, may experience disenfranchised grief when others perceive the child's death as a "blessing" rather than a loss for the family. Disenfranchised grief also occurs when bereaved persons are not recognized by society as capable of grief or needing to mourn. Young children, mentally challenged children or adults, and abusing parents whose actions have caused the child's death are often disenfranchised in this way.

Complicated or Troubled Grief

The processes of grief and mourning are normal and healthy aspects of human living. However, all human processes can go awry, especially in particularly difficult situations, and such grief is sometimes referred to as "complicated" grieving. As everyone who has experienced the loss of a loved one knows, all grief is complicated. It is just that sometimes grief is more complicated than at other times. Symptoms of complicated grief commonly include separation or traumatic distress, distinct from depression and anxiety.[9] Worden[10] has outlined four basic types of complicated grief: (1) chronic grief is characterized by grief reactions that do not subside and continue over long periods of time; (2) delayed grief is characterized by grief reactions that are suppressed or postponed, and the family member consciously or unconsciously avoids the pain of the loss; (3) exaggerated grief occurs when the family member resorts to self-destructive behaviors, such as suicide; and (4) masked grief occurs when the family member is not aware that behaviors that interfere with normal functioning are a result of the loss. Those who are mourning the loss of a child are at risk for complicated grief.

Factors Affecting the Grief Process

Individual Factors

History and Relationship With the Child
Each parent, sibling, or grandparent has a unique history and relationship with the deceased child. Histories among siblings are closely intertwined because siblings often develop special bonds that are unlike any other. The closer two siblings are to one another before death, the more behavior problems the

surviving sibling may have following the death.[11] Similarly, grandparents may be integrally involved in children's lives, whether they live geographically far apart or down the street; in other families, grandparents and children barely know one another. Some histories among the children and other family members will have been predominantly troubled (filled with tension and conflict) and others filled with laughter and harmony.

Previous Experience With Death

Past experiences with death and the learned response to loss also affect how each family member will grieve a child's death. Other deaths of a similar nature may have occurred in the family, such as when more than one child suffers from the same life-limiting genetic disorder. How previous losses were handled in the family will influence the current situation.

Developmental Level

When we think of "developmental level," we often think only of children and adolescents. Variants of four subconcepts of death are commonly included in writings about children and death: irreversibility, nonfunctionality, universality, and inevitability.[12] But development is a lifelong process; therefore, the developmental level of each grieving individual must be considered.

Young parents who are facing the death of their child have not typically experienced many life crises; elderly grandparents may be struggling under the burden of having faced too many. A teenage mother, struggling to be independent from her parents, faces new challenges when she must rely on them for assistance because her baby becomes ill and dies. A midlife father, anxious about his family's financial future following his son's long-term illness, agonizes deeply over the expenses of his son's funeral and feels guilty about his feelings. A grandmother who overcame breast cancer at age 65 years laments over why her 20-year-old granddaughter was the one to die from cancer.

Personality and Coping Style

Individuals of all ages vary in temperament and personality, and styles of interacting with the world are evident in even the youngest children. Some youngsters are naturally more extroverted; they talk easily with others and eagerly seek out resources and sources of support and comfort. Others are more introverted; they keep their thoughts and feelings to themselves and may prefer the solitude of reading or quiet play. Doka describes styles of grieving among adults that occur along a continuum, with "instrumental" grieving at one end and "intuitive" grieving at the other.[7] Most people fall in the middle, but describing the extremes of the continuum clarifies the differences and may be helpful in understanding how parents and other family members manifest their grief. Intuitive grievers fit the pattern of how we think individuals "should" grieve.

Environmental Factors

Role in the Family of the Child Who Died

Ordinal position often defines children's roles in the family. When a child dies, shifts occur among the other children. For example, Jose was the eldest of three sons. When he died, his father told Marco, the middle son, that he was now the "oldest." The three boys had shared very close relationships, and now the surviving two felt that their father was "forgetting" Jose by no longer regarding him as the eldest son. Children also play particular social, spiritual, and physical roles in the family; the child's absence leaves their role unfilled, and resultant adjustments can be difficult for remaining family members. Jose had been the "leader"; Marco did not want to assume his brother's leadership role. Also, how the child defined the other members of the family affects their grieving. Again, Jose particularly liked to joke about his "little" brother, who was growing to be taller than Jose. Marco had enjoyed the teasing and did not want to displace his admired older brother. Tension grew between father and sons.

Family Characteristics

Even before their child dies, families have characteristic ways of being in the world, of solving problems, of managing crises, of interacting with one another, and of relating to those outside the family. When a child is seriously ill and dies, families respond in the ways that are typical for how they manage other life events. These ways of coping are more or less functional. Earlier research with families of adult patients[13] and with pediatric patients[11] documented eight dimensions of family functioning: communicating openly, dealing with feelings, defining roles, solving problems, using resources, incorporating changes, considering others, and confronting beliefs. These dimensions occur along a continuum of functionality so that family interactions tend to vary along the continuum rather than being positive or negative, or good or bad.[11] The nurse's role is to assess each family's way of functioning and to realize that some families are more difficult to assess and work with than others. For example, some families may not wish to share information in the presence of their children, others do not wish to discuss matters with any relatives in the room, and still other families include everyone in most discussions. Thus, it is important for the nurse to gather information over time and to talk with more than one family member to appreciate the varied perspectives. Most families value the opportunity to tell their story, and thus listening becomes a central aspect of caring for grieving families.

Social and Cultural Characteristics

No one grieves in isolation from others. Friends, extended family, and community support influence how the family unit and individual family members function and come to terms with a child's death. A friend with a sensitive presence and listening ear can be of significant support to a grieving parent or sibling. Or, when grieving parents are challenged by the responsibilities of parenthood, a kind and supportive aunt or uncle can help to maintain a normal routine and a safe and understanding environment for the surviving siblings.

Individuals and families grieve within broader cultural contexts. Some turn to culture and tradition to find support and comfort in the answers, rituals, ceremonies, behavioral prescriptions, and spiritual practices they provide. Others do not strongly identify with the beliefs and mores of their cultures of origin, even when other members of their own family may do so.

Watching a child fall sick and die is a crisis of meaning for families, and it is through their cultural understandings and practices that families struggle to explain and make sense of this experience.[14,15] Spiritual or religious rituals may help families find meaning when their child dies. However, such rituals may interfere with the expression of grief if they prescribe, rather than foster creation of, meaning of the child's death for individual family members.

Situational Factors

Characteristics of the Child's Illness and Death

Where or when a child died, decision-making about the death, memories of sights and sounds, degree of medical intervention, and the cause of death are all subject matters that families discuss during bereavement while exploring their grief. Ideally, the location (home or hospital) of a child's death is based on the family's specific needs and requests, but circumstances (insurance issues, nursing shortages, transportation issues) may preclude achieving this goal. Long-term outcomes for bereaved parents and siblings of home care deaths suggest an early pattern of differential adjustment in favor of home care deaths.[16,17]

Decisions at the end of life, such as withdrawal of life support, may have been made with parents feeling they had insufficient understanding of the situation. Lasting images or smells may be comforting or concerning to families, depending on their associations. In fact, pain or other distressing symptoms the child might have experienced provide powerful material for families to struggle with during their grief. A full code that ends with the child's death is very different than if a child slips into death from an unconscious state. A child's death that follows years of treatment is experienced very differently from one that occurs quickly.

Involvement in the Illness and Death-Related Events

Growing consensus supports informing children about their medical condition and involving them in discussions and decisions about their care that are appropriate for their levels of cognitive and emotional maturity.[18] The same is true for involving siblings in the care of the ill child and in the events surrounding the death, such as the funeral, memorial service, and burial rituals. In one study, children who were more involved in such activities had fewer behavioral problems following the death.[11] At the same time, practitioners must consider not only the individual child's capacity for involvement but also the family's values about discussions of death, medical care, and children's roles.

Impact of Grief and Bereavement on Family Members

Dying Children

Children react to their own dying, as they do to most of life's experiences, within their cognitive and emotional capabilities. They live and die as children, but often with much apparent wisdom, sometimes seeming to surpass that of their adult caregivers. One of the earliest studies of seriously ill children indicated that very ill children are, indeed, aware of death and are more anxious than children hospitalized for nonserious illnesses or nonhospitalized children.[19] Bluebond-Langner,[20] based on her ethnographic study of dying children, subsequently described a process of how they become aware of their own impending death (Box 6.1). The children may experience a wide range of feelings, including but not limited to anger, anxiety, sadness, loneliness and isolation, and fear. Behaviors may include avoiding deceased fellow friends' names or staying away from their belongings; reducing attention to non–disease-related chatter and play; being preoccupied with death and disease imagery, particularly in play; engaging in open talk about the death only with selected persons; feeling anxious about weakened body functions and doubts about going home; evading talk of the future; being concerned with things being done right away; regressing, such as refusing to cooperate with relatively easy, painless procedures; or having estranged relationships with others, demonstrated by anger or silence.

This work provides some background for understanding terminally ill children, such as this 14-year-old boy whose death is imminent:

> My mother used to go to church to pray for me early every morning. I also prayed in my bed for my mother to stop her soundless sorrow. We were

---

Box 6.1 The Process of Children's Perceptions of Their Own Impending Death

1. I am ill. For some children there is a clear beginning to their illness, although there may be a gray period before their diagnosis. For others, with a progressive disease, the realization is likely to be more gradual but is eventually reached.

2. I have an illness that can kill people. Some children reach this stage simply because they hear a word like *leukemia* and know perhaps rather vaguely that it is associated with death. Others are told by their parents, if for no other reason than to help explain why the treatment given is so awful. The understanding that comes at this stage is virtually academic, and it is possible that some children do not believe what they are told.

3. I have an illness that can kill children. When there are three boys with cystic fibrosis in a school one summer term and only two in the autumn, the remaining two have had the clearest possible lesson. We should always be on guard for the ripples that come to a hospital ward or the school class when a death occurs.

4. I am never going to get better. This may follow on quite quickly after stage 3, or it may take some time. It is almost always associated with depression. This does not imply children know their death is imminent.

5. I am going to die. Some authors suggest that all children from 3 years and up are capable of reaching this stage. One must be open to the possibility that even very young children may have a full understanding not only of death but also of their own death.

Reprinted with permission from Goldman A. *Care of the Dying Child*. Oxford, New York: Oxford University Press; 1994. Reprinted with permission of Oxford University Press (UK).[21]

all sad and we pray separately in different places. Now, I am getting more worried about how sad she will be after my death, and she will feel lonely without me. How can I express my sorrow for her and thank her? She has lost so many things . . . money, time, and smiles, all because of me. . . .

Parents

Parent-child relationships are not contractual, but sacred. They are unique and complex. The connectedness between parent and child has its roots in the biologic and emotional bonds and attachments that precede birth. It grows as the parent begins to know and care for the child. The child is a parent's link to the future.[22] Parental grief is all-consuming, affecting every aspect of parents' existence. Parental bereavement after a child's death involves a level of suffering for both parents. Cacciatore, Erlandsson, and Rådestad[23] note that fathers' emotions are often overlooked in deference to the mother's grief. Yet fathers experience suffering and express gratitude, when nurses and others acknowledge their level of distress.

Parents often struggle with guilt following their child's death because of deep-rooted feelings of responsibility for their child's welfare. Because parents are responsible for protecting and sustaining their children, shielding them from all danger, many parents feel they should have protected their child from illness and death. When children die from an inherited disease such as cystic fibrosis or sickle cell anemia, parents know their child's condition results from their unknowingly passing on the genetic material. When the child dies, parents may still carry the burden of knowing they "gave" their child a terminal illness. Parents whose child died from an accident may also feel guilty for abdicating their protective role. Bereaved parents may cling to irrational guilt because it is often easier to accept blame, with its fantasy of control, than the total loss of control with which they must grapple. Or, they may blame someone else for their child's death. Sometimes this guilt is targeted toward a partner or spouse, another child, or a family member. Nurses need to be aware of these dynamics and help a family find an appropriate place for their anger and blame.[24] They may also adopt a stance of protecting the other parent from their own grief, paradoxically resulting in increased grief for both.[25] Nurses can help by acknowledging the "normality" of a variety of grieving styles and encouraging parents to understand each other's ways of grieving.

Nurses must also be cognizant of the special needs of bereaved parents who cope with additional stressors in their everyday lives. Single parents or same-sex parents may not have as many options for support as married parents in a heterosexual relationship. Moreover, nurses must pay attention to the indirect grief of parents who witness or coexperience the death of other terminally ill children in the same clinical setting as their child.[26]

Grandparents

The grief of grandparents is twofold: they have to bear their own grief, as well as bear the agony of the grief of their own child, the parent of the deceased child, a phenomenon termed "double pain."[27] In addition, grandparents experience "cumulative pain."[27] Gilrane-McGarry and O'Grady identified three sources in addition to the double pain: pain from their own past losses, pain common to all grief, and witnessing negative changes in their child. Grandparents identified two factors highly relevant to nursing care that helped them with their grief: having their loss acknowledged and being considered a part of the bereaved family.[28] Grandparents can be a source of considerable strength for parents and siblings, or they can be an additional source of stress. Their advice may be sought but then ignored; often their practical help is accepted, but their own grief is barely acknowledged. Extended family is a part of the child's team. Healthcare providers may be both challenged and gratified as they work to integrate their presence and ideas into palliative care practice and family support.[29,30] Grandparents may experience considerable helplessness and frustration; they question the meaning of life as they struggle with the "lack of order" of having the young one precede them in death.

Siblings

Siblings have been called the "forgotten grievers." They have been typically ignored when a brother or sister dies, not for lack of parental concern, but because their parents are so overcome with grief that they have little energy to devote to the needs of their surviving children. The impact of a child's death on surviving siblings is manifested in four general responses, best characterized in the words of the children themselves:[31] "I hurt inside," "I don't understand," "I don't belong," and "I'm not enough."

"I Hurt Inside"

The first response includes all the emotions typically associated with grief—sadness, anger, frustration, loneliness, fear, guilt, restlessness, and a host of other emotions that characterize bereavement. Unlike adults who are able to talk about their responses, children manifest their responses in various behaviors, such as withdrawing, seeking attention, acting out, arguing, being afraid to go to bed at night, overeating, or undereating. In response to children who are hurting inside, nurses need to allow, and even encourage, the expression of the hurt the children are feeling. They may endeavor to share their own thoughts and feelings with the children to let them know that they are not alone in this situation. If adults do not allow children to express their feelings, siblings learn there is something wrong with such feelings. When adults are impatient with children, or belittle their expression, siblings learn to stifle their feelings.

"I Don't Understand"

Children's difficulty in understanding death is greatly influenced by their level of cognitive development. However, once children know about death, their cognitive worlds are forever altered. If they are not helped to understand what has happened in clear, simple, and age-appropriate ways, children make up their own explanations that usually involve taking responsibility for the death and their parents' distress. Without explanations, they become more frightened and insecure. Nurses must have a solid grasp of children's cognitive development, provide appropriate explanations for events that happen, and be open to questions from children.

"I Don't Belong"

A death in the family tears apart the usual day-to-day activities and patterns of living. Parents are overwhelmed with their grief, with making arrangements, and with caring for their other children. Surviving children are overwhelmed with the flurry of activity and the depth of emotion surrounding them. They often feel as if they don't know what to do; they may want to help, but they don't know how, or, if they try, their efforts are not acknowledged. They begin to feel as if they are in the way, or as if they are not a part of what is happening. They feel different from their peers as well and begin to feel as if they don't belong anymore. Nurses can play a critical role in including siblings in illness and death-related events, such as encouraging or teaching the child to participate in certain treatments (e.g., by holding their sibling's hand or blowing bubbles together during painful procedures). After death, the nurse can help the parents by modeling what to say to the children.

"I'm Not Enough"

Assuming that they are somehow responsible for their parents' distress, siblings may feel as if they are not enough to make their parents happy ever again. They may feel that their deceased brother or sister was the favorite child and that they should have been the one to die instead. Some siblings respond by striving to be as good as they can be, trying to prove that they are worthy. They must be made to feel special just for being themselves and by not comparing them to their deceased brother or sister. Moreover, siblings may not want to burden their parents with their grief, knowing their parents are already overladen. Nurses can assist siblings to feel special by asking questions about their lives and reassuring them of their value and unique characteristics or abilities.

Adolescents

Teenagers who are dying or who are the siblings or friends of another child are often overlooked.[32] They face a particularly complicated situation when they encounter death and bereavement because adolescents are typically engrossed in achieving independence and in proving their invulnerability. Serious illness and grief catches them by surprise because they seldom have developed the coping skills necessary to deal with their reactions. As well, many adults believe it is difficult to help adolescents cope with death because adolescents are reputed to turn away from adults and to talk only with other adolescents. This is not entirely true; these young people often seek out and value the input and support of adults they respect, such as a teacher, a nurse, or a friend's parent. Moreover, when adolescents turn to their peers, if they do, they may often find that their peers have no significant resources to offer because they too are inexperienced with death.

Dying adolescents with a terminal disease struggle against physical pain, are sensitive to their parents' reactions, and have a strong desire to have relationships with their friends regardless of their illness status: "I couldn't say anything with my Mom. She pretends to smile to me, but I know how she feels so sad whenever looking at me. I want to come out and share my emotions with my friend at least. But, now there is nobody around me." In such cases, nurses are in a position to help an adolescent's family members to understand adolescent cognitive and psychosocial functioning. Self-help support groups for teens, either in person or on the Internet, often prove valuable to grieving adolescents. Adolescents are often open to writing, art, or music. Adults may come along on such journeys, or share the results, but they should take care to follow the adolescents' lead, respecting confidentiality and permitting them to interpret the significance of their work in their own way.

Assessing Grief

Grief assessment focuses on the ill child, other family members, and their significant others and it begins when the child is admitted to the hospital or at the time of diagnosis of acute, chronic, or terminal illness. It is ongoing throughout the course of the child's illness and comes to the forefront during the bereavement period after the death. As illustrated in Figure 6.1, an integrative model of bereavement care, as opposed to a series or parallel

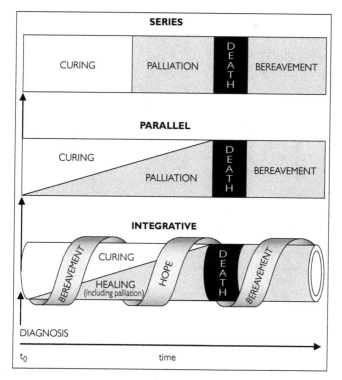

Figure 6.1. Integrative model of curing and healing (with bereavement and hope). Copyright 2010, Jay Milstein. Modified by Rana Limbo and Kathie Kobler. Used with permission.[33]

model, highlights the central role of bereavement support for a family from the moment they suspect their child is ill. Nurses, in particular, play a central role in a family's initial bereavement experience, holding in mind the family's sense of loss, while pursuing with other team members care that best addresses the child's well-being. Most children's deaths still occur in the hospital; nurses are most often present at the time of death. If not with the child at the moment of death, the nurse is usually the first one called to the child's bedside. The nurse's words and actions at that time leave indelible imprints on parents.

Helping Bereaved Families

Grief assessment leads to a plan of care with the goal of facilitating and supporting the grieving process. Understanding grief as a normal, human process that is individually expressed enables practitioners to present an accepting, nonjudgmental attitude that helps create a respectful and trusting milieu.

Grief Interventions

For Families

Bereaved individuals need an opportunity to express their grief in a supportive environment. Nurses have a responsibility to create such an environment for parents and other family members following a child's death so that they feel it is okay for them to express whatever they are feeling. Such comments as, "It must be very difficult for you right now" give permission for expression. The form of expression may vary among family members; some will verbalize, others will cry, some may leave the room. Still others may express anger, and others appreciation.

For Children

Grief is a human response, and children and adults alike feel denial, anger, sadness, guilt, and longing in response to death of a loved one, and they experience lack of sleep, lack of appetite, and difficulty concentrating and maintaining usual patterns of interaction with others. However, most children have limited ability to verbalize and describe their feelings; they also have very limited capacity to tolerate the emotional pain generated by open recognition of their loss.[33] Moreover, children's cognitive developmental level interferes with their ability to understand the irreversibility, universality, and inevitability of death and to understand their parents' reactions. They also deeply fear being different in any way from their peers and so are often unable to find comfort, as adults do, in sharing their discomfort with their friends. Because play is the work and the language of childhood, children are able to express their feelings through their play, as well as music and art. A summary of grief reactions in children, according to age level, and corresponding suggested interventions, is presented in Table 6.1.

Table 6.1 Grief and Bereavement in Children

Characteristics of Age	View of Death and Response	What Helps
Birth to 6 Months of Age		
Basic needs must be met; cries if needs are not met	Has no concept of death	Progressively disengage child from primary caregiver if possible.
	Experiences death like any other separation—no sense of "finality"	
Needs emotional and physical closeness of a consistent caregiver		Introduce a new primary caregiver.
	Nonspecific expressions of distress (crying)	Provide nurture and comfort.
		Anticipate physical and emotional needs and provide them.
Derives identity from caregiver	Reacts to loss of caregiver	
View of caregiver as source of comfort and all needs fulfillment	Reacts to caregiver's distress	Maintain routines.
Developing trust		
Age 6 months to 2 years		
Begins to individuate	May see death as reversible	Provide continual support and comfort.
Remembers face of caregiver when absent Demonstrates full range of emotions	Experiences bona fide grief	Avoid separation from significant others.
	Grief response only to death of significant person in child's life	Close physical and emotional connections by significant others.
Identifies caregiver as source of good feelings and interactions	Screams, panics, withdraws, becomes disinterested in food, toys, activities	Maintain daily structure and schedule of routine activities.
	Reacts in concert with distress experienced by caregiver	Support caregiver to reduce distress and maintain a stable environment.
	Has no control over feelings and responses; may display regressive behavior	Acknowledge sadness that loved one will not return; offer comfort.
Age 2 to 5 years		
Egocentric	Sees death like sleep: reversible	Remind child that loved one will not return.
Cause-effect not understood	Believes in magical causes	Reassure child that he or she is not to blame.

(continued)

Table 6.1 (Continued)

Characteristics of Age	View of Death and Response	What Helps
Developing conscience	Has sense of loss	Give realistic information and answer questions.
Attributes life to objects	Curiosity, questioning	Involve child in "farewell" ceremonies.
Feelings expressed mostly by behaviors	May display regression, clinging	Encourage questions and expression of feelings.
	Commonly displays aggressive behavior	Keep home environment stable and structured.
Can recall events from past	Worries about who will care for him or her	Help the child put words to feelings; reassure and comfort the child.
		Reassure the child about who will take care of him or her; provide ways to remember loved one.
Age 5 to 9 years		
Attributes life to things that move; may fear the dark	Personifies death as ghosts, "bogeyman"	Give clear and realistic information. Include the child in funeral ceremonies if the child chooses.
Begins to develop intellect	Is interested in biologic aspects of life and death	Give permission to express feelings and provide opportunities; reduce guilt by providing factual information. Maintain structured schedule and individual and family activities. The child needs a strong parent.
Begins to relate cause and effect; understands consequences		
	Begins to see death as irreversible	
Is literal, concrete	May see death as punishment; may feel responsible	
Has decreasing fantasy life, increasing control of feelings		
	Has problems concentrating on tasks; may deny or hide feelings, is vulnerable	Notify school of what is occurring; provide gentle confirmation and reassurance.
Preadolescence through teens		
Is undergoing individuation outside home	Views death as permanent	Provide unambiguous information.

(continued)

Table 6.1 (Continued)		
Characteristics of Age	View of Death and Response	What Helps
Identifies with peer group; needs family attachment	Sense of own mortality; sense of future	Provide opportunities to express self, feelings; encourage outside relationships with mentors.
	Strong emotional reaction; may regress, revert to fantasy	
Understands life processes; can verbalize feelings		
	May somaticize, intellectualize; may have morbid preoccupation	Provide tangible means to remember loved one; encourage verbal and nonverbal self-expression.
Is experiencing physical maturation		
		Dispel fears about physical concerns; educate about maturation; provide outlets for energy and strong feelings (e.g., recreation, sports); provide mentoring and direction.

Reprinted with permission from Fine P, ed. *Processes to Optimize Care During the Last Phase of Life*. Scottsdale, AZ: Vista Care Hospice; 1998.[34]

For Parents

Before the child's death, an important emphasis for clinicians is to facilitate connections between the parents and the ill child and their other children, as well as to help them develop memories and keepsakes that they can hold and cherish long after the death. The earlier these can be collected, the better, so that they reflect a longer period of time with the child and not simply the final days of life. Facilitating communication between family members and the caregiving staff, as well as among family members themselves, also creates positive memories and optimal coping. Informing parents about the dying process and helping them with the concept of appropriate death consistent with patient, family, cultural, and spiritual goals are necessary. Assisting with planning funeral or memorial services also can be helpful, particularly for families who have limited support systems.

After the child's death, follow-up by the clinicians who cared for the child is much appreciated by families. Such follow-up also allows ongoing assessment (see Box 6.2 for questions to ask during an initial follow-up telephone call). Parents, overcome with their own grief, may need assistance in dealing with the needs of their other children; encourage parents to enlist the support of aunts, uncles, or good friends in this regard. For parents who are willing and

Box 6.2 Questions for an Initial Follow-up Telephone Call to Parents Who Have Experienced the Loss of a Child or Perinatal Loss

- "You might recall that you were told that someone from the hospital would call you in (number) weeks."
- "Is this a good time to talk?"
- "Are there any issues that you have been thinking about that perhaps I could follow-up on for you?"
- "Have you been back yet for a post partum checkup?"
- "Some parents have noticed a change in their sleeping or eating habits. Has this been a problem for you?"
- "How has (name of other parent) responded to your loss? Sometimes it is hard for both parents to talk about it. How has it been for you?"
- "Do you have other family members or friends that you have been able to talk to? What types of things have they been able to do for you?"
- "Do you have plans to work outside of your home? The first few days at work can be especially difficult. Have you thought about how it might be for you?"
- "Did you receive any information on support groups for parents?"
- "Are there any other materials you received in the hospital that you have questions about?"
- "Are there any other questions I can answer for you?"
- "During the call you stated that. . . ."
- "I will call you again on (date)."

Reprinted with permission from Friedrichs J, Daly MI, Kavanaugh K. Follow-up of parents who experience a perinatal loss: facilitating grief and assessing for grief complicated by depression. *Illness Crisis Loss.* 2000;8(3):302.[35]

interested in finding additional support, provide a listing of parental support groups and other parent bereavement resources in the community, such as Compassionate Friends, a self-help organization to help parents and siblings after the death of a child (www.compassionatefriends.org).

Bereavement Programs

A bereavement program within pediatric palliative care, or as part of an agency-wide program, can be of considerable service to both families and staff. These services typically include staff with specific training in bereavement care and a follow-up component.[36] A bereavement program facilitates family referrals to grief therapists as needed; ensures that all families are made aware of the available services, such as support groups, memorial services, or grief workshops; and may facilitate bereaved families' connecting with one another as a source of support.

The Nurse: Suffering, Cumulative Loss, and Grief

Professionals who help children and families with the serious illness and death of a child are witness to numerous heart-wrenching scenes and are constantly reminded of the frailty and preciousness of life. Working with dying children can trigger nurses' awareness of their own personal losses and fears about their own death, the death of their own children, and mortality in general. Historically, nurses and other healthcare professionals were taught to desensitize themselves to these experiences and maintain an "emotional detachment." This approach, which still exists today in many situations, results in the nurses' use of defenses to allay their fears, including focusing only on physical care needs, evading emotionally sensitive conversations with children and families, and talking only superficially about topics that are comfortable for the nurse. These behaviors result in emotional distancing, avoidance, and withdrawal from dying children and their families at a time when children most need intensive interpersonal care and active involvement by the nurse. Death anxiety occurs when clinicians are confronted with fears about death and have few resources or support systems to explore and to express thoughts and emotions about dying and death.[36] Thus, rather than a "desensitization" of oneself, professionals are encouraged to sensitize to this powerful human material. Caring for dying children requires nurses to explore, experience, and express their personal feelings regarding death. Personal death-awareness activities and exercises, discussion of belief systems about death and afterlife with friends and colleagues, self-exploration, and reflection may promote an understanding and acceptance of death as part of life. The process is complicated by cumulative loss—a succession of losses experienced by nurses who work with patients with life-threatening illness and their families, often on a daily basis.[37,38] When nurses are exposed to death frequently, they seldom have time to grieve one child before another child dies.

In addition to helping bereaved families, as mentioned earlier, institutional bereavement programs also serve the needs of staff. Programs can be structured to offer help in debriefing after a death, validating staff feelings, offering support groups, and encouraging informal support through the one-one-one sharing of experiences with coworkers, peers, or pastoral care workers[39,40] (Box 6.3). In addition, nurses can serve vital roles in co-creating ritual for both families and professional caregivers. The presence of a supervisor, mentor, or instructor during the care of the dying, when a family member visits, or during the time of the child's death can greatly decrease anxiety and provide immense support to the nurse, particularly to novice nurses in pediatric palliative care.

Pediatric palliative care is a challenging field, one that demands finding the balance between providing compassionate quality care and personal satisfaction as a professional nurse. In addition, working with dying children and their families provides meaning to life. Working with these children helps nurses to develop a clear perspective of what is really valuable; it helps us grow

Box 6.3 The Challenges of Educating Healthcare Professionals

Challenge 1: Develop a philosophy of teaching that promotes relational learning and reflective practice.

Challenge 2: Develop curricula that include goals, learning objectives, and methods of teaching that focus on relationships with the dying, the bereaved, and coworkers.

Challenge 3: Integrate current knowledge into educational programs and supervised clinical applications.

Challenge 4: Evaluate training outcomes as well as the context and process by which learning occurs.

Challenge 5: Integrate formal and informal learning activities into the work context.

Reprinted with permission from Papadatou D. *In the Face of Death.* New York: Springer; 2009.[36]

as persons and professionals. From the children and their families, we learn that death is part of life, human beings are remarkably resilient, and hope is everlasting.

References

1. Field MJ, Behrman RE; Institute of Medicine (US) Committee on Palliative and End-of-Life Care for Children and Their Families. *When Children Die: Improving Palliative and End-of-Life Care for Children and their Families.* Washington, DC: National Academies Press; 2003.

2. Meert KL, Briller SH, Schim SM, et al. Examining the needs of bereaved parents in the pediatric intensive care unit: a qualitative study. *Death Stud.* 2009;33(8):712-740.

3. Hexem KR, Miller VA, Carroll KW, et al. Putting on a happy face: emotional expression in parents of children with serious illness. *J Pain Symptom Manage.* 2013;45(3):542-551.

4. Gilmer MJ, Foster TL, Vannatta K, et al. Changes in parents after the death of a child from cancer. *J Pain Symptom Manage.* 2012;44(4):572-582.

5. Rando TA. *Clinical Dimensions of Anticipatory Mourning: Theory and Practice in Working With the Dying, Their Loved Ones, and Their Caregivers.* Champaign, IL: Research Press; 2000.

6. Rando TA. *Grief, Dying, and Death: Clinical Interventions for Caregivers.* Champaign, IL: Research Press; 1984.

7. Doka KJ. *Disenfranchised Grief: Recognizing Hidden Sorrow,* Lexington, MA: Lexington Books; 1989.

8. Doka KJ. *Disenfranchised Grief: New Directions, Challenges, and Strategies for Practice.* Champaign, IL: Research Press; 2002.

9. Lobb EA, Kristjanson LJ, Aoun SM, et al. Predictors of complicated grief: a systematic review of empirical studies. *Death Stud.* 2010;34(8):673-698.

10. Worden JW. *Grief Counseling and Grief Therapy: A Handbook for the Mental Health Practitioner.* New York, London: Springer; 2008.

11. Davies B. *Shadows in the Sun: The Experiences of Sibling Bereavement in Childhood*. Philadelphia, PA: Brunner/Mazel; 1999.

12. Hunter SB, Smith DE. Predictors of children's understandings of death: age, cognitive ability, death experience and maternal communicative competence. *Omega (Westport)*. 2008;57(2):143-162.

13. Davies B. *Fading Away: The Experience of Transition in Families with Terminal Illness*. Amityville, NY: Baywood Publishing; 1995.

14. Kenner C, Boykova M. Palliative care in the neonatal intensive care unit. In: Ferrell B, Coyle N, eds. *Oxford Textbook of Palliative Nursing*. 3rd ed. New York: Oxford University Press; 2010:1065-1080.

15. Boss R, Kavanaugh K, Kobler K. Prenatal and neonatal palliative care. In: Wolfe J, Hinds PS, Sourkes BM, eds. *Textbook of Interdisciplinary Pediatric Palliative Care*. Philadelphia, PA: Elsevier/Saunders; 2011:387-401.

16. Vickers J, Chrastek J. Place of care. In: Goldman A, Hain R, Liben S, eds. *Oxford Textbook of Palliative Care for Children*. Oxford, UK: Oxford University Press; 2012:391-401.

17. Dussel V, Kreicbergs U, Hilden JM, et al. Looking beyond where children die: determinants and effects of planning a child's location of death. *J Pain Symptom Manage*. 2009;37(1):33-43.

18. Hinds PS, Oakes LL, Furman WL. End-of-life decision-making in pediatric oncology. In: Ferrell B, Coyle N, eds. *Oxford Textbook of Palliative Nursing*. New York: Oxford University Press; 2010:1049-1064.

19. Klass D, Silverman PR, Nickman SL. *Continuing Bonds: New Understandings of Grief*. Washington, DC: Taylor & Francis; 1996.

20. Bluebond-Langner M. *How Terminally Ill Children Come to Know Themselves and Their World*. Princeton, NJ: Princeton University Press; 1978:166-197.

21. Goldman A. *Care of the Dying Child*. Oxford, New York: Oxford University Press; 1994.

22. Arnold JH, Gemma PB. *A Child Dies: A Portrait of Family Grief*. 2nd ed. Philadelphia, PA: Charles Press; 1994.

23. Cacciatore J, Erlandsson K, Rådestad I. Fatherhood and suffering: a qualitative exploration of Swedish men's experiences of care after the death of a baby. *Int J Nurs Stud*. 2013;50(5):664-670.

24. Worden JW, Monahan JR. Caring for bereaved parents. In: Armstrong-Daily A, Zarbock S, eds. *Hospice Care for Children*. 3rd ed. New York: Oxford University Press; 2009:181-200.

25. Stroebe M, Finkenauer C, Wijngaards-de Meij L, et al. Partner-oriented self-regulation among bereaved parents: the costs of holding in grief for the partner's sake. *Psychol Sci*. 2013;24(4):395-402.

26. James L, Johnson B. The needs of parents of pediatric oncology patients during the palliative care phase. *J Pediatr Oncol Nurs*. 1997;14(2):83-95.

27. Gilrane-McGarry U, O'Grady T. Forgotten grievers: an exploration of the grief experiences of bereaved grandparents (part 2). *Int J Palliat Nurs*. 2012;18(4):179-187.

28. Gilrane-McGarry U, O'Grady T. Forgotten grievers: an exploration of the grief experiences of bereaved grandparents. *Int J Palliat Nurs*. 2011;17(4):170-176.

29. Davies B, Orloff S. Bereavement issues and staff support. In: Hanks G, Cherny NI, Christakis NA, et al., eds. *Oxford Textbook of Palliative Medicine*. 4th ed. Oxford, New York: Oxford University Press; 2009:1361-1372.

30. Friebert S, Chrastek J, Brown MR. Team relationships. In: Wolfe J, Hinds PS, Sourkes BM, eds. *Textbook of Interdisciplinary Pediatric Palliative Care*. Philadelphia: Elsevier/Saunders; 2011:148-158.

31. Marshall B, Davies B. Bereavement in children and adults following the death of a sibling. In: Neimeyer RA, ed. *Grief and Bereavement in Contemporary Society: Bridging Research and Practice*. New York: Routledge; 2011:107-116.

32. Balk DE. Sibling bereavement during adolescence. In: Balk DE, Corr CA, eds. *Adolescent Encounters With Death, Bereavement, and Coping*. New York: Springer; 2009:199-216.

33. Milstein J. A paradigm of integrative care: healing with curing throughout life, "being with" and "doing to." *J Perinatol*. 2005;25(9):563-568.

34. Fine P, ed. *Processes to Optimize Care During the Last Phase of Life*. Scottsdale, AZ: Vista Care Hospice; 1998.

35. Friedrichs J, Daly MI, Kavanaugh K. Follow-up of parents who experience a perinatal loss: facilitating grief and assessing for grief complicated by depression. *Illness Crisis Loss*. 2000;8(3):302.

36. Papadatou D. *In the Face of Death: Professionals Who Care for the Dying and the Bereaved*. New York: Springer; 2009:330.

37. Kobler K, Limbo R. Making a case: creating a perinatal palliative care service using a perinatal bereavement program model. *J Perinat Neonatal Nurs*. 2011;25(1):32-41.

38. Vachon MLS, Huggard J. The experience of the nurse in end-of-life care in the 21st century: mentoring the next generation. In: Ferrell B, Coyle N, eds. *Oxford Textbook of Palliative Nursing*. New York: Oxford University Press; 2010:1131-1156.

39. Keene EA, Hutton N, Hall B, Rushton C. Bereavement debriefing sessions: an intervention to support health care professionals in managing their grief after the death of a patient. *Pediatr Nurs*. 2010;36(4):185-189.

40. Rushton CH, Reder E, Hall B, et al. Interdisciplinary interventions to improve pediatric palliative care and reduce health care professional suffering. *J Palliat Med*. 2006;9(4):922-933.

Index

A

Academy of Neonatal
Nursing, 94
acetaminophen, 30*t*, 59–60,
85*t*, 114
adjuvant analgesics, 59,
63, 114
Adolescent Pediatric Pain
Tool (APPT), 55*t*
adolescents, impact of grief
on, 130–31
advanced childhood illness
assessing sources of
suffering, 25, 27–28
expectations and goals of
care, 27–28
illness
experience, 25, 27
Aging With Dignity, 17
agitation
causes of, 38*b*
children with advanced
disease, 37–38
management of, 39*t*
albuterol, 43*t*
American Academy of
Pediatrics, 1, 83
American Pain Society, 51
anemia, 26*b*, 29*b*, 30*t*
anesthetic
techniques, 63–64
anorexia
children with advanced
disease, 28*b*, 34–35
factors contributing
to, 35*b*
management of, 36*t*
anticipatory grief, 122
anxiety
children with advanced
disease, 28*b*, 35–36
suffering, 13
Association of Women's
Health, Obstetric and
Neonatal Nurses, 94
atropine, 34*b*
authorized agent-controlled
analgesia (AACA), 63
autopsy
child's death, 116–17
neonatal end of life
care, 91

B

Baptist, influence on
care, 76*t*
beliefs about pain,
open-ended
questions, 14*t*
bereavement
children, 133–35*t*
helping families in, 132
impact on family
members, 126–31
integrative model of
curing and healing, 131*f*
pediatric palliative
care, 21
programs, 136
see also grief
Buddhist, influence on
care, 76*t*
burns, pain, 49

C

cachexia
children with advanced
disease, 34–35
factors contributing
to, 35*b*
management of, 36*t*
cancer, pain, 50–51
carbamazepine, 41*t*
cardiovascular
conditions, 26*b*
caregivers, hospice
care, 81*b*
Centering Corporation, 94
Center to Advance Palliative
Care (CAPC), 22
children
adolescents and
grief, 130–31
assessment of
pain, 56, 58
bereavement, 133–35*t*
care at time of
death, 17–18
communicating about
integrating palliative
care, 100–101*t*
complex chronic
conditions, 26*b*
death in the
home, 18–20*b*

development stages, 3*t*
grief interventions, 132,
133–35*t*
identification for
hospice and palliative
care, 6–8
impact of grief on
dying, 126–28
intensive care unit
(ICU), 99–100,
105, 107
needs for life-threatening
illness, 7*f*
pain-related
developmental
milestones, 52–56*t*
perceptions of
own impending
death, 127*b*
rituals celebrating child's
life, 115–16
Children's Health Insurance
Program (CHIP), 4
Children's Hospital of
Eastern Ontario Pain
Scale (CHEOPS), 53*t*
chronically ill children, 7,
37, 101–2
Church of Jesus Christ
of Latter-Day Saints
(Mormon), influence on
care, 76*t*
clonazepam, 39
clonidine, 64, 85*t*
COMFORT scales, 113
communication
compassionate,
effective, consistent
bidirectional, 107–10
effective, with
families, 108
end of life family
conferences, 108
having difficult
discussions, 106–7*b*
integrating palliative
care, 100–101*t*
medical decision-
making, 109–10
methods for sensitive
healthcare
information, 103–5*t*

communication (*Cont.*)
open-ended
questions, 14–15*t*
palliative care, 11–12
post-death
conference, 117
strategies for improving
team, 108
complex chronic conditions,
childhood, 26*b*
complicated grief, 123
concurrent care, 2, 4
*Concurrent Care for Children
Implementation
Toolkit*, 4
constipation
children with advanced
disease, 28*b*,
31–32
intensive care unit
(ICU), 114
management of, 33*t*
critical care
extubation
technique, 112
forgoing no-longer
beneficial
interventions, 112–13
transfer to alternative
care settings, 112–13
cultural beliefs, palliative
care, 13, 16
cultural care, palliative
care, 12
cultural practice, death of
child at home, 20
cultural sensitivity, neonatal
end of life palliative
care, 92
culture, influences on
care, 73–75

D
death
autopsy and organ
donation, 116–17
care at the time
of, 17–18
emergency or
ICU personnel
communicating, 102,
105
epidemiology of
pediatric, 97
integrative model
of curing and
healing, 131*f*
notification in ED and
ICU, 116
perceptions of, 3*t*
post-death
conference, 117

see *also*
bereavement; grief
death rattle, 42, 115
decision-making
child participation
in, 101–2
end of life, 110
medical, 109–10
depression, 13, 28*b*, 37
developmental
milestones,
pain-related, 52–56*t*
dexamethasone, 32*t*
dextroamphetamine, 30*t*
diarrhea
children with advanced
disease, 28*b*, 33–34
management of, 34*b*
diazepam, 39, 41*t*, 86*t*
diphenhydramine, 30*t*, 39*t*
diphenoxylate, 34*b*
disenfranchised grief, 123
District of Columbia
Pediatric Palliative Care
Collaborative, 4
do-not-resuscitate (DNR)
order, 27, 90, 102, 110
dronabinol, 36*t*
ducosate sodium, 33*b*
dyspnea
causes of, 42*b*
children with advanced
disease, 40–41
intensive care unit
(ICU), 114–15

E
education
healthcare
professionals, 138
pediatric palliative
care, 22
Educational
Development Center
(EDC), 22
emergency department
(ED), 97
acute unexpected illness
or injury, 98
aggressive symptom
management
in, 113–15
effective communication
with families, 108
needs of parents of
ill/injured children
in, 98–99
notification of death
in, 116
palliative care
consideration
in, 98–100

personnel communicating
news of
death, 102, 105
emergency kit, 8
emotional issues,
open-ended
questions, 14*t*
emotional support, 12
end of life
decision-making, 110
family
conferences, 108
management of
seizures, 41*t*
recommendations and
implementation, 118
see *also* neonatal end of
life palliative care
End-of-Life Nursing
Education Consortium
(ELNEC), 22, 83, 94
Epidemiology, pediatric
death, 97
Episcopal, influence on
care, 77*t*
ethical principles
pediatric palliative
care, 16–17
perinatal palliative
care, 74*t*
extubation, 112

F
family
communicating about
integrating palliative
care, 100–101*t*
communication
with healthcare
team, 11–12
core concepts of family
care, 75*b*
death of child at
home, 18–20*b*
end of life
conferences, 108
grief interventions, 132
hospice care, 81*b*
impact of grief and
bereavement
on, 126–31
intensive care unit
(ICU), 105
neonatal end of
life palliative
care, 86, 91–92
family dynamics, advice from
parent, 10*b*
fatigue
children with advanced
disease, 28*b*, 29
management of, 30–31*t*

feeding problems, 34
fentanyl, 60t, 61t, 62t, 85t
first responders, 8
Five Wishes (for adults), 17, 102
FLACC (Face, Legs, Activities, Cry and Consolability), 113

G

gastrointestinal symptoms, 26b, 28b
anorexia and cachexia, 34–35, 35b, 36t
feeding problems and intolerance, 34
genetic conditions, 26b
glycopyrrolate, 31, 43t, 86t
goals of care, advanced childhood illness, 27–28
grandparents, impact of grief on, 128–29
grief
anticipatory, 122
assessing, 131–32
complicated or troubled, 123
disenfranchised, 123
environmental factors, 124–26
factors affecting process, 123–26
impact on family members, 126–31
individual factors, 123–24
interventions, 132–36
nurse, 137–38
pediatric palliative care, 21
as process, 121
situational factors, 126
types of, 122–23
see also bereavement
guardians, support for, 9–10

H

haloperidol, 39t
healthcare information, methods for communicating sensitive, 103–5t
healthcare professionals
challenges of education, 138
communication with team, 11–12
respecting parents' wants and needs from, 8

hematologic and immunodeficiency conditions, 26b
Hindu, influence on care, 78t
hope, preserving, 16
hospice agencies, 5, 6t
Hospice and Palliative Nurses Association (HPNA), 22
hospice care
availability, 5, 6t
definition and evolution of, 2
newborns/infants and adults, 75, 81b
human immunodeficiency virus (HIV), 26b, 33, 49, 51
hydromet (combination of hydrocodone and homatropine), 43t
hydromorphone, 43t, 62t
hyoscyamine, 43t

I

ibuprofen, 59t, 60t
Initiative for Pediatric Palliative Care (IPPC), 22
Institute for Patient- and Family-Centered Care, 75b, 95
Institute for Safe Medical Practices, 63
intensive care unit (ICU), 97
acute unexpected illness or injury, 98
aggressive symptom management in, 113–15
child participation in decision-making, 101–2
children with chronic life-threatening conditions in, 99–100
considering suffering and quality of life, 110–11
constipation, 114
continuity and coordination of care needs, 101–2
dyspnea, 114–15
effective communication with families, 108
end of life decision-making, 110
end of life family conferences, 108
forgoing no-longer beneficial interventions, 111

medical decision-making, 109–10
needs of child in, 107
notification of death in, 116
pain, 113–14
palliative care consideration in, 98–100
palliative sedation, 115
patient and family needs in, 105
personnel communicating news of death, 102, 105
strategies for improving team communication, 108
interdisciplinary team (IDT), 2
pediatric palliative care, 8–9
psychological symptoms and suffering, 12–13
International Society for Krishna Consciousness, influence on care, 78t
interventions
grief, 132–36
palliative care, 7f
intolerance, 34
Islam (Muslim/Moslem), influence on care, 77t

J

Jehovah's Witnesses, influence on care, 78t
Judaism, influence on care, 78t

L

local anesthetics, 63–64, 113–14
logistics, palliative care, 7f
loperamide, 34b
lorazepam, 30t, 39, 39t, 85t
Lutheran, influence on care, 79t

M

McCaffery, Margo, 47
magical thinking, 54t, 55t
malignancy, 26b
management, pain, 58–64
mechanical ventilation, 41–42
Medicaid, 2, 4
Medicare, 2
megestrol, 36t
metabolic conditions, 26b
methadone, 62t, 85t

Methodist, influence on care, 79t
methylphenidate, 30t
metoclopramide, 31, 32t
midazolam, 30t, 85t
Mormon, influence on care, 76t
morphine, 43t, 60t, 61t, 62t, 85t, 112, 114
My Wishes (resource for young children), 17, 102

N

National Association of Neonatal Nurses (NANN), 82, 95
National Board for Certification of Hospice and Palliative Nurses (NBCHPN), 22
National Hospice and Palliative Care Organization (NHPCO), 2, 4, 5, 6t, 22
nausea
   children with advanced disease, 28b, 31
   management of, 32t
neonatal end of life palliative care
   autopsy suggestions, 91
   cessation of aggressive support, 90–91
   environment for neonatal death, 88–89
   family care, 91–92
   family follow-up care, 92
   introducing model to parents, 87–88
   location for provision of, 89–90
   medications, 85–86t
   newborn categories, 87
   ongoing staff support, 92–93
   organ and tissue procurement, 91
   pain and symptom management, 90
   planning, 84
   prenatal discussion, 84, 86
   protocol, 84–93
   ventilator removal, 90
Neonatal Facial Coding System, 53t
Neonatal Infant Pain Scale (NIPS), 52t
neonatal intensive care unit (NICU), 69, 83–84

advocacy for support, 82–83
case study, 69–72
new trends, 83
neonatal patients
   advocacy for support services, 82–83
   cultural influences on care, 73–75
   differences in palliative care, 75, 81b, 82
   family as unit of care, 73
   palliative care medications, 85–86t
   palliative care plans, 82
   religious influences, 73–75, 76–80t
   standard of care for, 72–73
neurodegenerative disorders, 26b
neurologic
   symptoms, 26b, 28b
   restlessness and agitation, 37–38, 38b, 39t
   seizures, 38–39, 40b
neuropathic pain, 49
nociception, 47
nonopioids, pain, 59–60
nonpharmacologic management, pain, 64
nurses
   pediatric palliative care, 21–22
   suffering, cumulative loss and grief, 137–38

O

ondansetron, 32t
opioids, pain management, 60–62
organ donation
   child's death, 116–17
   neonatal end of life care, 91
outpatient pediatric palliative care, 5, 6t
oxycodone, 61t
oxymorphone, 62t

P

pain
   assessment in children, 56, 58
   barriers to pain control, 57–58t
   burns, 49
   cancer, 50–51
   definitions of, 47
   emergency department and ICU, 113–14

etiology of, in children, 49–51
human immunodeficiency virus (HIV) infection, 51
improvement areas, 65
management, 58–64
neuropathic, 49
nonpharmacologic management, 64
pain-related developmental milestones, 52–56t
pharmacologic management, 58–64
physiology and pathophysiology of, 51, 56
prevalence in children, 47, 49
procedural pain management, 64–65
questions for evaluating children with, 48–49t
sickle cell disease, 51
pain management, 12, 58–64, 90
paracetamol, 59t, 60t
parents
   assessing psychosocial concerns and strengths, 14–15t
   death of child at home, 18–20b
   grief interventions, 135–36
   impact of grief on, 128
   introducing palliative care model to, 87–88
   questions for follow-up call after loss of child, 136b
   suddenly ill/injured children in emergency department, 98–99
   support for, 9–10
patient-controlled analgesia (PCA), 63
Patient Protection and Affordable Health Care Act (PPPACA), 4
patients
   assessing psychosocial concerns and strengths, 14–15t
   core concepts of care, 75b
   hospice care, 81b
   review of care plan, 111
pediatric hospice, 1
pediatric palliative care (PPC)
   anticipatory grief and bereavement, 21

availability, 5, 6t
care at time of
death, 17–18
communication, 11–12
comparing PPC and
hospice care, 2
comprehensive
assessment, 12
creating a sacred
space, 18, 20
definition of, 1–2
education and
training, 22
essential elements in, 7f
ethical
considerations, 16–17
healthcare
professionals, 137–38
identifying children
for, 6–8
interaction with
schools, 11
interdisciplinary team
(IDT), 8–9
needs for life-threatening
illness, 7f
nursing care issues
for, 21–22
pain and symptom
management, 12
preserving hope, 16
psychological symptoms
and suffering, 12–13
religious, spiritual,
and cultural
considerations, 13, 16
respecting parents' wants
and needs, 8
self-care, 21
setting for, 4–5
support for parents and
guardians, 9–10
support for
siblings, 10–11
target group for, 5f
see also bereavement;
grief; physical
symptoms
Pentecostal
influence on care, 79t
perinatal palliative care
ethical principles and
application, 74t
support and
providers, 8, 9f
pharmacologic
management
pain, 58–64
phenobarbital, 39, 41t
phenytoin, 41t
physical symptoms
advanced and terminal
disease, 28b, 28–29

anxiety, 28b, 35–36
constipation, 28b,
31–32, 33t
depression, 28b, 37
diarrhea, 28b, 33–34, 34b
fatigue, 28b, 29, 30–31t
feeding problems and
intolerance, 34
nausea, 28b, 31, 32t
vomiting, 28b, 31, 32t
physicians
neonatal end of life
palliative care, 86
post–death conference, 117
post–traumatic
stress disorder
(PTSD), 105, 109
practical issues
open–ended
questions, 15t
Premature Infant Pain Profile
(PIPP), 113
prenatal discussion
palliative care, 84, 86
Presbyterian
influence on care, 80t
procedural pain
management, 64–65
promethazine, 32t
psychological support, 12
psychological symptoms and
suffering, 12–13
psychosocial concerns and
strengths, open-ended
questions for, 14–15t

Q

Quakers, influence on
care, 77t
quality of life, considering
future, 110–11
questions
assessing psychosocial
concerns and
strengths, 14–15t
follow-up call for
parents with loss of
child, 136b
QUESTT approach, pain
assessment, 58

R

religion
death of child at
home, 20
influences on neonatal
care, 73–75, 76–80t
palliative
care, 12, 13, 16
renal conditions, 26b
Resolve Through Sharing
(RTS) Bereavement
Training, 95

respiratory
symptoms, 26b, 28b
dyspnea, 28b, 40–41
management of, 43t
mechanical ventilation in
PPC, 41–42
terminal respirations, 42
restlessness
causes of, 38b
children with advanced
disease, 37–38
management of, 39t
rituals, celebrating child's
life, 115–16
Roman Catholic, influence
on care, 74, 80t

S

schools, interaction
with, 11
sedation, palliative, 115
seizures
children with advanced
disease, 28b, 38–39
management of, at end of
life, 41t
patterns in children, 40b
self-care, pediatric palliative
care, 21
senna, 33b
siblings, impact of grief
on, 129–30
sickle cell disease
(SCD), 26b, 49,
51, 128
social support, 12
Society of Friends, influence
on care, 77t
spiritual beliefs, palliative
care, 12, 13, 16
spiritual needs, open-ended
questions, 15t
staff support, neonatal
end of life palliative
care, 92–93
sudden infant death
syndrome
(SIDS), 97, 118
suffering
assessing sources of, in
advanced childhood
illness, 25, 27–28
considering, 110–11
Sumner, L. H., 18–20b
support services, advocacy
for, 82–83
symptom management
aggressive, in ED and
ICU, 113–15
neonatal end of life
care, 90
palliative care, 12

T

terminal respirations, 42
tissue procurement,
        neonatal end of life
        care, 91
training, pediatric palliative
        care, 22
transport issues,
        neonatal end of life
        palliative care, 86–87
troubled
        grief, 123

U

Unspoken Grief, 95

V

ventilator removal, neonatal
        end of life care, 90
Voicing My Choices (for
        adolescents), 17, 102
vomiting
    children with advanced
        disease, 28b, 31
    management of, 32t

W

World Health Organization
        (WHO), 1, 50, 59t,
        60t, 61t, 62t
www.agingwithdignity.
        org, 17

Z

zolpidem, 30t

CPSIA information can be obtained
at www.ICGtesting.com
Printed in the USA
LVHW020512280720
661655LV00014B/1725